Lifelong Le   ing

PREP in

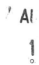

Maggy Wallace

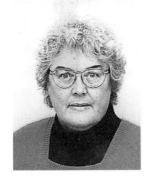

Maggy Wallace is an independent consultant and author working in the field of professional standards and development. She is a registered nurse, teacher and librarian, with a background in nursing practice, education and policy making. She has a particular interest in continuing professional development. She directed the implementation of the PREP project at the UKCC, where she worked for a number of years in a range of senior positions, most recently that of Director of Standards Promotion. She left to pursue an independent career in 1997. Since then she has, together with her UK work, undertaken a number of overseas assignments, including consultancy for the World Health Organization. She is on the International Council of Nurses' Expert Panel on regulation and has represented the ICN in an expert capacity. She has also worked with other health professionals in the UK on continuing professional development and competency issues.

She lives in the country near Watership Down, with her husband, dogs (3 at the last count), friends and other animals. Her husband, daughter and son-in-law are all teachers – her son is still fighting his inevitable destiny.

Dedication

For my friends and colleagues, past and present, who really understand what professional regulation is about.

For Churchill Livingstone:

Senior commissioning editor: Alex Mathieson
Project manager: Ewan Halley
Project controller: Derek Robertson

Lifelong Learning
PREP in action

Maggy Wallace MA BA RN DipN RCNT DipEd RNT
Independent Consultant, formerly Director of Standards Promotion, UKCC

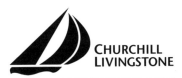

CHURCHILL
LIVINGSTONE

EDINBURGH LONDON NEW YORK PHILADELPHIA SYDNEY TORONTO 1999

CHURCHILL LIVINGSTONE
An Imprint of Harcourt Brace and Company Limited

Churchill Livingstone, Robert Stevenson House, 1–3 Baxter's Place,
Leith Walk, Edinburgh EH1 3AF, UK

First published 1999

ISBN 0 443 06142 4

British Library Cataloguing in Publication Data
A catalogue record for this book is available from the British Library.

Library of Congress Cataloging in Publication Data
A catalog record for this book is available from the Library of Congress.

The
publisher's
policy is to use
**paper manufactured
from sustainable forests**

Printed in China
EPC/01

Contents

Preface

I have enjoyed writing this book and I hope you will enjoy reading it. I know that a lot of nurses, midwives and health visitors are worried about meeting their requirements for continuing professional development – known as PREP. This book tries to make sense of the PREP requirements and to reassure those who are concerned that they are achievable.

More importantly, the book puts all of the PREP activity into context and shows how changes to the ways in which we work and the move to lifelong learning, in particular, are influencing us all. These changes are particularly relevant for the health care professions as we continually strive to improve the standard and quality of care that we give to those who depend upon our expertise at a time when they are at their most vulnerable. Although written mainly with nurses, midwives and health visitors in mind, the book will have considerable relevance for other professional colleagues.

I hope that the book will give you plenty to think about and that you will feel refreshed and enthused after reading it – excited at the prospect of a future that you are helping to shape.

Acknowledgements

I would like to thank all those friends and colleagues who have both inspired and in some way contributed to this book – whether it has been in the interest that they have shown, their help in retrieving both knowledge and information, in their comments on early drafts or providing coffee when necessary.

Although I cannot mention everyone by name, as there are too many, Heather Williams and Reg Pyne must be identified, as their prodigious memories and generous spirits have sustained me throughout. I would also like to thank Bernie O'Connell and Catherine Jenkins for their help and interest – past and present.

And finally, to Les, Kate, Jamie and my father, who are always there for me.

A map of the world that does not include Utopia is not worth even glancing at, for it always leaves out the one country at which Humanity is always landing. And when Humanity lands there, it looks out and seeing a better country sets sail.

The Soul of a Man under Socialism, Oscar Wilde

Introduction

Nothing in education is so astonishing as the amount of ignorance it accumulates in the form of inert facts.
(*The Education of Henry Brook Adams*, Henry Brook Adams)

WELCOME

I hope you are going to enjoy owning, or, at the very least, reading this book. I can promise you that it certainly will not be an accumulation of inert facts. Henry Brook Adams clearly had a bad educational 'experience'.

I know that there is a real tendency to skip over the introduction in books – I do it myself. But could I ask you to make an exception in this case, because to make sense of the book and get the best out of it, it really would be very helpful to read this part. Who knows, you may even enjoy it?

This book is really two books in one – how about that for value for money? There is, as you would expect from the title, comprehensive detail about the requirements for maintaining and developing professional knowledge and competence, which are now an essential part of registration as a nurse, midwife or health visitor. These requirements, as many of you will know, are known colloquially as 'PREP', which stands for post-registration education and practice. The book not only gives you details of the actual requirements (which you can also find elsewhere), but also tells the unique story, which has not been told before, of how the PREP project came into being and how the requirements were developed and agreed. This is a unique part of the profession's history and is a story which deserves to be told. Equally important, but probably far less well known to many readers, is the wider context within which these changes were made – in other words, the lifelong learning movement, the changing ways of work and the developing emphasis on continuing professional development (CPD).

This book will contain quite a lot of facts – after all, I have no doubt that that is why you are reading it – but they will be relevant, easy to understand

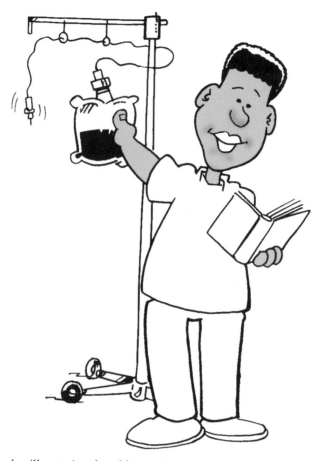

'The book will contain a lot of facts – but relevant, easy to understand and applicable to your situation.'

and applicable to your current situation, whether you are working at the moment, having a break for any reason, or considering possible future career options. What it will do is to set out for you, in a clear and readable way, the statutory requirements for re-registration. In other words, it describes the PREP requirements, simply, clearly and, I hope, reassuringly. More importantly, I believe, it will help you understand how all these changes came to be made and how they are part of the wider context of lifelong learning, continuing professional development and changes to the ways in which society is organizing its patterns of work.

So it is not just a mechanical regurgitation of the facts which you can already read about in the useful information provided by organizations such as the United Kingdom Central Council for Nursing, Midwifery and Health Visiting (henceforth – you will be relieved to hear – to be known as the

UKCC or the Council), e.g. in the *PREP fact sheets* (UKCC 1994) or the *PREP and You* booklet (UKCC 1997). It is more than that. It will also help you to consider the wider aspects of your professional development, both now and for whatever your future may hold.

So, what is the book about, who is it for, why has it been written, why have I written it, and why should you invest your time and effort in reading it?

What is the book about?

At the risk of insulting some of my readers, I think I do need to reiterate very clearly what has already been said about the content of the book. And I do this, regrettably, on the basis of very recent evidence that came to me towards the end of 1997, whilst this book was in preparation. At a large conference held for registered practitioners (nurses, midwives and health visitors) in London, one of the speakers was taken severely to task by someone in the audience for 'using jargon'. The 'jargon' in question was the words 'the UKCC'. Perhaps I shouldn't be surprised, as there are over 640 000 registered nurses, midwives and health visitors in the UK, but I – and many of my colleagues present at the event in question (some of whom were not themselves nurses, midwives or health visitors) – was surprised. After all, who are we all actually registered *with*??

So. At the risk of offending some, I am going to quickly state the bald facts. The United Kingdom Central Council for Nursing, Midwifery and Health Visiting (snappy little title, isn't it?) is the statutory, regulatory body set up by an Act of Parliament to set standards for professional education and conduct for nurses, midwives and health visitors. To practise as a nurse, midwife or health visitor in the UK, you *must* be registered with the UKCC.

In 1995, new requirements relating to maintaining your registration, known as the PREP requirements, came into force for all nurses and health visitors, together with changed requirements for midwives. These new requirements related to keeping up-to-date by undertaking study activity, keeping a personal professional profile and doing return-to-practice courses if you had had a break in practice. If the requirements are not met, then your registration will lapse and you will not be eligible to practise your profession.

This book looks at all these issues in detail.

Who is the book for?

The book is intended to be relevant to *all* nurses, midwives and health visitors who are currently registered with the UKCC or who have been registered in the past but whose registration has lapsed and who are considering whether it is worth the effort of re-registering. In 1997 there were over 640 000 of us on the UKCC's professional register – an enormous professional group consisting of about 36 000 practising registered midwives, 24 000 registered health visitors and the rest nurses. Health visitors, remember, always qualify first as nurses, which explains the convention that I will use throughout the book, in which I will always talk about nurses and midwives when I am referring to everyone on the register. This is accurate and shorter and is certainly not intended to offend health visitors.

There are 15 parts to the UKCC's register, the parts 'being indicative of different qualifications and different kinds and standards of training' (Section 7, The Nurses, Midwives and Health Visitors Act; HMSO 1997). Although you don't need to know the parts by name, it is just worth reminding ourselves how varied they are, particularly the nursing qualifications. As it is easier to do this by parts of the register, I have used this as the framework. Broadly, for nursing, there are two levels of qualification – first and second – in a variety of different nursing fields. Midwifery is more straightforward, as is health visiting.

Part 1 (SRN RGN RN). This is by far the largest part of the register, as it is the part for first level 'general' nurses. It includes those whose original qualification was that of state registered nurse (SRN) as well as those who qualified more recently and use the title registered general nurse (RGN). Many individuals now just use the title registered nurse (RN), which is, of course, perfectly acceptable. Individuals on this part of the register will have qualified by a variety of means. The majority will probably have completed a 'traditional' 3 year course, which was very much an apprenticeship style training. Others will have done one of the 'experimental' courses, such as that known as the '2 plus 1' course (which was a 2 year education programme followed by 1 year under supervision as a staff nurse). Some will have completed a nursing qualification together with a degree, in either nursing or a related subject. Yet others will have done a post-registration course of 18 months or 2 years, following a previous registration. A few will have undertaken a 'shortened' course, by virtue of a degree in another subject.

Part 2 (EN(G)). This is the part of the register for second level (or enrolled) nurses, who have undertaken their 'general' training. It will include, in the main, those who completed a 2 year, or less, mainly practical training in general nursing, with assessments and examinations. There are, however, still a few enrolled nurses who were 'enrolled' by means of experience, although these numbers are, understandably, now very few.

All 'enrolled' nurses can, of course, refer to themselves appropriately as registered nurses, as their names appear on the UKCC register.

Part 3 (RMN). This is the part of the register for those with a first level qualification in psychiatric or mental nursing. Although the numbers are not so large, the ways in which those registered here obtained their qualification will be very similar to those on Part 1.

Part 4 (EN(M)). This is the part for second level nurses who have undertaken their qualification in psychiatric or mental health nursing. Routes to obtaining the qualification will be similar to those on Part 2.

Part 5 (RNMH RNMD RNMS). This is the first level part of the register for those qualified in what is now known as learning disabilities nursing, but which over time has been known variously as mental handicap, mental deficiency or mental subnormality nursing. Its registrants will have similar qualification patterns to those on Part 3 and Part 1.

Part 6 (EN(MH)). This is the second level part of the register for those referred to in Part 5.

Part 7 (EN). This is the part of the register for those individuals who did a generic course, usually 18 months in length, in Scotland or Northern Ireland. Employment would be in the field of practice in which they have had the majority of their experience, so it could be in general, mental health, learning disabilities or, rarely, children's nursing.

Part 8 (RSCN). Sick children's nurses are registered in this part, either as a result of a 3 year course, or more often, as the result of a 4 year combined course leading to registration as both a general and a children's nurse. Occasionally, the qualification was achieved post-registration. There are no second level parts of the register for children's nurses, although some nurses who qualified on Part 7 may be employed in this field.

Part 9 (RFN). I doubt if many readers realize that there is still a part of the register for fever nurses but that's what this part refers to – registered fever nurse. There are still some individuals on the register who are practising by virtue of their RFN qualification alone, but as training ceased in the 1960s, they are, not surprisingly, rapidly diminishing in number.

Part 10 (SCM RM). All registered midwives are registered on Part 10 of the register. The majority will have undertaken a shortened post-registration qualification, following an initial qualification as a nurse. However, there are increasing numbers who are undertaking the midwifery qualification as a first qualification, following a 3 year programme, and practising solely as a midwife.

Part 11 (RHV). Part 11 is for registered health visitors. All health visitors have to qualify initially as nurses before undertaking a programme of an academic year in length to qualify as a health visitor.

Parts 12, 13, 14 and 15. Individuals on these parts of the register will have completed a Project 2000 programme. This will have consisted of a common foundation programme, 18 months in length, followed by an 18 month branch programme in their particular area of clinical practice. Their academic qualification will be no less than a higher education diploma. Registration will be in one of the following:

- adult nursing (Part 12 (RN))
- mental health nursing (Part 13 (RN))
- learning disabilities nursing (Part 14 (RN))
- children's nursing (Part 15 (RN)).

So, as you can see, our range is enormous. And the differences don't end with the parts of the register and the routes used to get registered. Some individuals on the register have undertaken no study since their original qualification; others have hardly stopped. Similarly, some people may have practised in one or more areas of nursing, midwifery or health visiting since they qualified. On the other hand, others may have had long periods out of practice for a whole variety of reasons – family commitments, unemployment, ill health or alternative careers. There will, indeed, be some who have never practised at all since qualification, including those who never got round to registering in the first place before going off and doing something else.

As you can see, there is a vast and diverse actual and potential professional workforce. Yet we are all united in one thing. *If we wish to be employed or to work as a registered nurse, midwife or health visitor, then we must be registered with the UKCC.* If we are to be registered, then we must meet the statutory requirements for registration. These statutory, or legislative, requirements are colloquially known as the 'PREP requirements' – PREP standing for post-registration education and practice. It describes the framework for maintaining and developing professional knowledge and competence, for renewing registration and for specialist practice.

So, I hope you are convinced – this book is for you. Indeed, I hope that it will also be of interest to other professions. Nursing, midwifery and health visiting have led the way within the health-related professions, and more widely, in terms of putting into place continuing professional development (CPD) requirements for all those who are practising or intending to practise. Our experience will, I am sure, be of help to those professions that are now considering systems of their own.

Why has the book been written?

The book has been written to fulfil a need. A large number of words have been written about PREP. In addition to the material put out by the UKCC, there have been lots of articles and explanatory material put out by other individuals and other organizations, particularly those providing continuing education materials. PREP has had its supporters, who have thought the whole idea was wonderful, and its detractors, who thought it was ill-conceived. Reassuringly, there have been very few of the latter, although there are those who 'wouldn't have done it this way'. Amidst it all stands *you*, the individual practitioner, trying to sort out the facts from the fallacies, the accurate from the inaccurate, the objective picture from the vested interests. As well as worrying about what it all means for you as an individual registered nurse, midwife or health visitor, you've probably also been trying to do your job, look for one if you haven't got one, pay the mortgage or rent, plan your future and cope with the vast amount of change being flung at you from all directions. Never has the phrase 'the only certainty is uncertainty' been more accurate.

Why have I written this book?

Simply, because I believe that I am in a unique position with regard to PREP. Let me explain. I had the privilege of working at the UKCC from 1985 to 1997. The word 'privilege' is not used lightly. I thought it was indeed an honour to be able to work for the one body in the UK which is required by its legislation, and in the public interest, to set standards for nursing, midwifery and health visitor education, practice and conduct. The key to the Council's standard-setting work is the professional register. All the UKCC's activity is targeted towards making the register the ultimate instrument of public protection.

There are three basic sets of standards:

- standards for entry on to the register
- standards for remaining on the register
- standards for removal from the register.

The work of the Council is, therefore, or should be, central to the essence of nursing, midwifery and health visiting.

I began life at the Council as professional adviser, listening to the problems and enquiries that practitioners were facing on a daily basis – problems with issues in professional practice, with terms and conditions of service, with relationships with colleagues, both from the same and from other professions, and with issues about confidentiality, accountability, ethics and career moves, to name but a few.

I then worked for a while as professional officer, nursing. This was at the time of the tail-end of the initial work on Project 2000, which was setting out proposals for a radical reform of nursing and midwifery education, to prepare for a move forward into the 21st century. I arrived just as the new proposals were being 'sold'. It was an exciting time, with Council members and officers travelling around the UK talking to a vast range of people about the proposed reforms – both employers who were able to 'cascade' the information down to their staff, and a wide range of representative and interested individuals from nursing, midwifery and health visiting, as well as from other professions. All this experience subsequently proved vital when the PREP work began.

At the end of 1989, the UKCC started to plan its major project on post-registration education and practice, which became known as PREPP (Post Registration and Education Practice Project). The project was initially directed by the UKCC's deputy registrar, Heather Williams, and I was the deputy director. Concurrently, I was also appointed, in 1990, to the new post of 'assistant registrar, education and registration'. In 1993, I took over the directorship of PREPP and took it through to its final policy position in March 1994, including the preparation of the relevant legislation to make it a statutory reality. Then on to implementation during 1994 and 1995. This included the final policy initiatives, e.g. those in relation to specialist practice and the 'transitional arrangements'. I then took up a new post at the UKCC in 1996, as director of standards promotion. Until I left the Council in April 1997, I continued to monitor the progress of PREP and had started to prepare the ground for the systems of effective evaluation.

I think it fair to say – without wishing to overstate the case – that PREP has been one of my passions! I truly believe that the vision of the UKCC, in putting into place flexible, innovative standards which enable practitioners to maintain and develop their professional knowledge and competence showed wisdom well in advance of that seen at the time in any other professions. The subsequent interest shown by other professions has indeed supported that view. So there you have it – as the author I am totally biased, but extremely well informed! I hope that this combination will make for interesting reading and that you will enjoy adding to your own knowledge.

What is in the book?

The information in this book is a mixture of things, and, indeed, is probably at least two books in one. There are the facts which you would expect, about the details and actual requirements of PREP, but there is much more than that. The whole PREP initiative is set into context against the broader canvas of lifelong learning, CPD and professional regulation. It addresses the responsibilities which lie with all professionals, in terms of maintaining their professional knowledge and competence. There is also the, as yet untold, story of the actual development of the PREP proposals and how they were influenced during the discussion and consultation processes by individual nurses, midwives, health visitors, employers, professional organizations and other professional colleagues, to name but a few.

Your contribution to the book

Most importantly, I believe, the book is brought to life by the experiences of people like yourselves, the readers. As you can imagine, over the past few years I have spoken to literally thousands of nurses, midwives, health visitors and others about the PREP proposals. Small groups in screened off side-wards, large groups in huge auditoria, worried individuals on the phone, delegates at professional organisation conferences, midwives doing refresher courses, groups in the NHS, groups in the independent sector – in registered nursing homes, residential homes, social service departments, independent hospitals, prisons; to mental health, learning disability, children's, community and general/adult nurses; to health visitors, managers, employers, chief nurses, students; doctors, physiotherapists, managers, pharmacists, GPs; practice nurses, occupational heath nurses... I could go on and on. The message, however, is simple. You have helped me to write this book and your

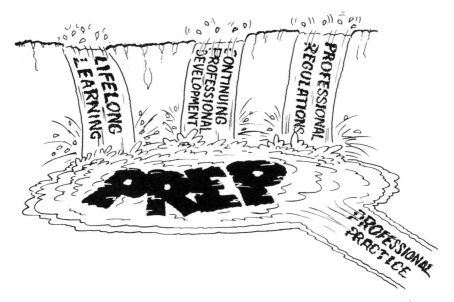

*'The PREP initiative is set into context against the broader canvas of lifelong
learning, continuing professional development and professional regulation.'*

experiences are here. It is your experiences, difficulties, challenges and,
above all, solutions which, I believe, make the book so relevant.

The other source of information about PREP issues has been the UKCC's
PREP helpline. The helpline was established in April 1995, at the UKCC, and,
as you would imagine, has been busy since it began. Questions about study
activity, funding, time off, professional portfolios, return to practice
programmes, notification of practice forms, notification of intention to
practise for midwives, 'approved' courses, and many others, come in on a
daily basis. The calls are all regularly logged and policies re-examined, to see
if any additional material needs to be provided, or any other type of changes
made.

The view from a distance

Possibly one of the greatest advantages, for the reader, of me writing this
book is that I have now left the UKCC. One of the things which becomes
immediately apparent once 'outside' the organization is the sheer difficulty
of obtaining reliable information about the Council's activities, in a clear,
readable format, which gives all the facts without sounding pompous and
'statutory body-ish'. Not all practitioners read the professional press – and
if they do, as the honest ones will tell you, it is only to look for new jobs or
to see if there is any scandal brewing. And anyway, the Council does not get
wide publicity, unless there has been a Council meeting or there has been a

particularly contentious professional conduct decision. The other written material which comes out of the Council, whilst often very good and informative, can only too easily get lost amongst the plethora of stuff vying for our attention as we all go about our daily business. Many people get to the various 'meet the UKCC' events throughout the UK, but even so, they are only a handful of those on the register.

So, having your own personal source of information, which you can annotate, stick additional bits of information in, keep by your personal professional profile (more of that later), will, I hope, be really useful. I also suspect that for many of us, a book is still the format we would choose for this type of information, even if the information may also come in electronic form.

How to use the book

There is no right or wrong way of using the book. You can read it from beginning to end, if that is how you like to read books. That would make sense because that is how it is designed – so that one chapter flows into another.

It starts with a look at lifelong learning in general (Ch. 2). This chapter then goes on to look at the changes in the world of work and explores what implications these changes and the impact of lifelong learning have on CPD.

The following chapter (Ch. 3) starts to focus more specifically on the nursing, midwifery and health visiting professions and explores the changing face of professional regulation and the implications of regulating individuals who are professionally accountable. These two chapters provide the backdrop and context for change. Chapter 4 looks at the origins, role and functions of the UKCC, which you will find helpful reading before moving on to Chapter 5, which tells the story of the PREP project. This is the first time that the story has been told and, as such, describes an important part of the profession's history. The next chapter is the one that probably caused you to buy – or at least read – the book, as it is here that the PREP requirements are described in detail (Ch. 6). The flexibility of the requirements are explained and a lot of myths are debunked. Specialist and advanced practice is dealt with separately, together with principles and practicalities of credit accumulation and transfer schemes (CATS) and the accreditation of prior (experiential) learning (AP(E)L) (Ch. 7).

The final chapter looks at the way forward for you as an individual. It looks at all the things that we all have to consider when planning our own professional goals and will probably be particularly helpful to those who are coming to this fairly new. However, I hope that it will also contain some new insights even for those who have been here before.

Appendix 1 will probably be a popular place for a lot of readers, so my 'guinea pigs' tell me, as it raises all the questions that you have always wanted to ask about PREP but didn't like to. Don't worry, now someone has – and the answers are there too! Appendix 2 deals with sources of information – where to go to find out about all that is on offer. Appendix 3 gives real life examples of how some people are meeting their PREP requirements. Sensible, workable, cheap suggestions are put forward for you to think about and to perhaps use for yourself.

However, if you don't like reading books from one end to another, that's fine. Each chapter can be read as a separate entity and is designed to be comparatively free-standing. So, for example, if all you are interested in to start with is whether you understand the actual requirements of PREP properly, then you only need to read Chapter 6. If all you want to know about is how the policy came into place then go to Chapter 5. However, I hope that you will want to do more than that. PREP is not an isolated phenomenon – it is part of a much wider movement of lifelong learning and continuing professional development and can only be understood properly if seen in this context. It is also much easier to understand the requirements, if you have looked at their background.

And next?

So, I have set myself the challenge of readability, clarity, comprehension and no pomposity! Only you can judge the success with which I have achieved those objectives. Please read on and then let me know if I've succeeded or not. You can contact me via the publishers.

REFERENCES

UKCC 1994 PREP fact sheets. UKCC, London
UKCC 1997 PREP and YOU. UKCC, London
HMSO 1997 The Nurses, Midwives and Health Visitors Act. HMSO, London *This Act, which was basically a consolidation Act, amalgamated the requirements of The Nurses, Midwives and Health Visitors Act of 1979 and The Nurses, Midwives and Health Visitors Act of 1992. The 1997 Act has differently numbered sections from the two previous Acts, which may cause some confusion to the reader who is familiar with the previous sources.*

2

Lifelong learning and continuing professional development

Certainty is out. Experiment is in.

(Handy 1995)

INTRODUCTION

Two thousand years ago, Heraclitus reminded those fortunate enough to listen to him that you could never step into the same river twice – it was forever changing, as was life. And we think the idea of lifelong learning is new!

This chapter looks at the whole concept of lifelong learning, the changes in the world of work and their relevance to continuing professional development (CPD). It traces the origins of the lifelong learning movement and considers the implications that the changes may have for all of us. It also looks at the impact of the movement on the professions in general, and the nursing, midwifery and health visiting professions in particular.

If I may be permitted a small digression…if you haven't read the introduction (Ch. 1) to this book – and I know that lots of people, myself included, have a tendency to turn straight to the first chapter – could I ask you to take a few minutes to go back and read it? It really will help to make sense of the rest of the book and put all of the contents into context.

A word of explanation to avoid confusion may be helpful at the beginning of this chapter. There will be numerous references to higher education throughout the book in general, but this chapter in particular. You will quickly notice that there is a deliberate assumption on my part that what is relevant to higher education is relevant to the nursing, midwifery and health visiting professions. I don't raise the issue in order to apologize, of course, but to make sure that I don't lose those individuals who think that, because their original training did not take place in higher education, they can – or, indeed, have to – dismiss what is being said as irrelevant to them. Let us have none of the 'Oh well, I haven't got a degree and am not one of these academic nurses/midwives/etc. etc., so this doesn't apply to me'. It *does* apply to you because you are a registered nurse, midwife or health visitor, a professional and an accountable practitioner. Education for our professions now takes place in higher education and those coming onto the register will have been educated in that environment. This should pose no threat to existing professionals who have acquired their experience over years of practice – this serves to complement the knowledge and skills of newer colleagues. We are all professionals and all of us on the register – however we got there – need to engage in the lifelong learning debate in one way or another. Please read on!

WHAT IS LIFELONG LEARNING?

There are probably many people who have heard the term 'lifelong learning'. However, there are probably not many who would be confident that their understanding of the term is the same as everyone else's – or even whether it's composed of two words or three! And what about all the other words that are used that apparently mean the same thing? Where do continuous development, continuing education, continuing professional development, continuing vocational education, permanent education, self-directed learning, lifelong education, recurrent education and the learning society all fit? Let's have a look at what has been said about them by various commentators. The first thing that will probably strike you is that this debate is not new, and the second is that not everyone agrees with each other's interpretation of events. This is unlikely to come as a surprise to you, I'm sure.

Let's start with my favourite definition of lifelong education. Pucheu (1974) describes it – lifelong education, that is – as 'an elastic concept meaning whatever the person using it wants it to mean'. I think that's tremendously reassuring and means that none of us can be wrong – always a good situation to be in. However, there are those who would think that I am ducking the question if I stop there, so let's look a little further. Lifelong education has also been described as 'a utopian idea whose main function is to stimulate people to think critically about education' (Ruegg 1974). This is a good description, combining the practical reality of having to give education serious thought with the concept of always striving for something better.

Two of the most interesting and influential writers on the subject are Professors Christopher K. Knapper, from the University of Waterloo, Canada, and Arthur J. Croxley, from the University of Hamburg. In the fly-piece to the second edition of their book *Lifelong Learning and Higher Education* (Knapper & Croxley 1991), they say 'to cope with the demands of a rapidly changing world, people must be capable of taking the initiative for their own education, and be motivated to continue learning throughout their lives'.

They identify a number of factors in the history of the development of life-long learning which are helpful in understanding how and why the movement had developed. Although their background is higher education, the issues they identify have great transferability. The issues discussed have particular relevance as we move on, in due course, to look at PREP within the wider context of lifelong learning – which is, after all, probably why you are reading this book. They identify the following factors as contributing to the move for lifelong learning:

- *changed learning needs* – with more people wanting to learn different things
- problems with *financing* – reduced funding, demands for more things and a need to make more effective use of resources
- increased concerns about *democratization and fairness* – the elimination of socioeconomic, gender and geographic inequalities
- a perceived need for *closer ties to day-to-day life* – harmonizing education and culture, relating education to work, linking education to peace and preservation of the ecosystem
- a call for *changed teaching and learning strategies* – flexible and democratic educational planning, provision of learning networks, more self-direction in learning.

All these things, originally identified in the 1970s and 1980s, have a very familiar ring to them, don't they? It was E. Faure and colleagues (Faure 1972) who started the debate in the early 1970s and indeed there was a Lifelong Learning Act passed in the United States as early as 1976. Initially, however, the term, particularly in the US, related in the main to what would probably be referred to in the UK as adult education. In Europe, more generally, the term lifelong learning became more frequently associated with the notion of linking learning and work. At a UNESCO Meeting of Experts in 1983, lifelong education was described as education for 'liberation, self-realization and self-fulfilment'.

In his book *Education and Politics in the 1990s – Conflict or Consensus*, Denis Lawton (1992), former director of the Institute of Education at the University of London, looks at the history of general education in England. He describes the 1944 Education Act as a 'consensus approach as part of a desire for a better, fairer world after World War Two'. In his view, this was never entirely achieved. The years between 1944 and 1979 were spent modifying the 1944 consensus and 'education became an area of drift rather than direction'. From 1979, he believes, a new conservative vision began to emerge, which was not based on consensus but was 'impoverished and socially divisive and potentially destructive' in that it focused mainly on the relationship between school and work, at the expense of school and the community. He believes that the ensuing Education Act of 1984 was born out of a spirit of conflict 'with a demoralized and defeated teaching profession in the background'. Gradually, however, he describes the emergence of a 'new' approach to what is called variously lifelong education, permanent education and the learning society. Although the names differ, the principles are the same, in that we are to think of education as a lifetime process, from the cradle to the grave, and involving all people.

Rather more prosaically, in 1984, the University Grants Committee (Madden & Mitchell 1984) defined continuing education as 'any form of education, whether vocational or general, resumed after an interval following the end of continuous initial education'. The phenomenon increasingly has a European dimension. The European Universities Continuing Education Network (EUCEN) has identified the following types of continuing education (1992):

- education for full-time mature students
- usual adult education
- part-time degrees and diploma post-experience vocational education courses, including staff development
- open access courses.

Many will be aware that 1996 was designated as the European 'year of lifelong learning' and a wide range of events took place around that year to promulgate the idea of the learning society and the need to continually add to our store of knowledge and skill for those working in the European Economic Area.

Sir Christopher Ball, chairman of the Higher Education Funding Council, says this, in *Learning Pays* (Ball 1991), about the learning society:

...the idea of a learning society offers a broad vision. It rejects privilege – the idea that it is right for birth to determine destiny. It transcends the principle of meritocracy, which selects for advancement only those judged worthy and rejects as failures those who are not. A learning society would be one in which everyone participated in education and training (formal or informal) throughout their life. It would be a society characterized by high standards and low failure rates.

There is an interesting connection made by some commentators between the total quality movement and lifelong learning. In *Total Quality in Higher Education – Continuous Development*, Lewis & Smith (1991) are of the view that:

...practitioners of total quality and the academy also share a belief in the need for continuous improvement. The academician may identify it as continuous learning or research, but for both, it is a belief in learning appropriate concepts, processes and skills and applying these skills to appropriate problems and projects.

The learning society comes back into focus in Sir Ron Dearing's seminal report (and the Garrick Report in Scotland) on higher education, *Higher Education in a Learning Society* (National Committee of Inquiry into Higher Education 1997). The following visionary objectives are set out for higher education:

- to inspire and enable individuals to develop their capabilities to the highest potential throughout life, so that they grow intellectually, are well equipped for work, can contribute effectively to society and achieve personal fulfilment
- to increase knowledge and understanding for their own sake and to foster their application to the benefit of the economy and society
- to serve the needs of an adaptable, sustainable, knowledge-based economy at local, regional and national levels
- to play a major role in shaping a democratic, civilized, inclusive society.

Although there are those who would disagree with some of the fundamental changes proposed in the Dearing report, I believe that very few people would disagree with his objectives for higher education. And central to those objectives, and indeed explicit within the title, is the concept of the learning society. The sense that you get when reading the objectives is one of continuous forward movement, that we should always be learning and striving to use our knowledge not only for our own personal fulfilment but also for the greater good of society. Such sentiments will, I am sure, resonate with those reading this book.

CHARACTERISTICS OF LIFELONG LEARNING

The literature gradually builds up a picture of a number of trends which contribute to the concept of lifelong learning. These include:

- an expansion of educational services outside the 'normal' school age – both before the conventional start of education and after it has ended
- an awareness, acceptance and embracing of the idea that 'learning' doesn't stop at the end of 'formal or statutory' education
- a greater interest in education and learning as a means of improving the quality of life
- an enhanced awareness of the relevance and applicability of education to the demands of day-to-day life, rather than as a separate or isolated entity
- an increased realization that specific job skills have a tendency to become obsolete very quickly
- an increased greater participation in decisions about education by a greater number of people, including parents, members of the public and consumers of education – both adults and children.

There are also a number of characteristics which have been attributed to lifelong learning itself. Knapper & Croxley (1991) identified the following:

- it is *intentional* – learners are aware that they are learning
- it has a definite *specific goal* and is not aimed at vague generalizations such as 'developing the mind'

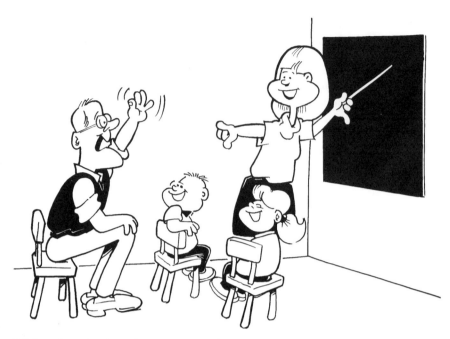

Lifelong learning is … 'an expansion of educational services outside the "normal" school age – both before the conventional start of education and after it has ended.'

- the goal is the *reason why* the learning is undertaken (i.e. it's not motivated by, for example, boredom)
- the learner intends to *retain* what has been learned for a long time (i.e. it is not spontaneous, unplanned or unconscious learning).

CHARACTERISTICS OF LIFELONG LEARNERS

Knapper & Croxley (1991) go on to say that the lifelong learner:

- is strongly aware of the relationship between learning and real life
- is aware of the need for lifelong learning
- is highly motivated to carry on lifelong learning
- possesses a self-concept favourable to lifelong learning
- possesses the necessary study skills.

Are you starting to recognize yourself yet? If you're not, you should be, or you wouldn't be reading this book.

What else do you need to be a lifelong learner? These are discussed in much more detail in the final chapter of this book, but they include skills like the ability to:

- *assess* your own personal and career needs, or at least find someone who can help you to do so

- *plan* your own realistic goals
- *implement* an effective action plan which helps you to achieve your goals
- *evaluate* the effect of your plan as it rolls out, modifying it as necessary.

Is this all beginning to sound familiar? It certainly should be. The process approach, which you will have met in the nursing process – love it or hate it – is an extremely effective 'coat hanger' for this type of activity.

IMPACT ON EDUCATION PROVIDERS

It almost goes without saying that if education 'consumers' were starting to think along the lines set out above, then there were going to be new and different demands on the providers of education, whether that was in schools, further education, higher education or the workplace.

You might like to reflect on some of the changes that may be taking place where you live, even if you had not consciously thought about them before. For example, do the local schools play a greater part in the life of the community now, e.g. as the venue for a range of activities, which may include use of the school facilities and may even involve the teachers themselves as well? Indeed, the issue of links with the community is now one of the areas subject to scrutiny in the visits by Ofsted inspectors.

Have you looked at the brochure of your local further education college(s) lately? If not, I would suggest that you do so, even if you think you have no spare time for anything else at the moment. The range of things that are on offer is truly amazing – ranging from taught courses for certificated subjects, such as GCSE or A levels, through to every imaginable 'leisure pursuit' such as car maintenance, calligraphy or quilt making. They also offer an interesting selection of health-related subjects, including the complementary therapies, such as aromatherapy or shiatsu. The type of courses range from an afternoon's 'taster' event to see whether you might be interested in studying the subject, through to 2 year courses demanding a regular and sustained commitment, with assessment and certification at the end. It is also interesting to look at the times when these events are offered. Practically any time of day or evening and Saturdays – I haven't seen anything on a Sunday yet but that is probably only because I haven't looked in the right place.

Higher education has had to respond even more dramatically to cope with the increasing demands of students who now expect and, indeed, demand a 'good' educational experience (Hazelgrove 1994). If they don't get it then they take their business elsewhere. This is true of all students now coming into higher education, but particularly so if we remain focused on our main area of interest – lifelong learners. If you think about the needs of that group, then it is fairly easy to start to compile a list of all the things that will need modification or change to meet the demand for a different type of educational experience.

Probably the biggest change that has been seen is in attitude to learning and the whole experience of higher education (Barnett 1989, 1992, Hazelgrove 1994) – of both students and teachers. Students bring the money with them and are a valuable commodity, and their 'business' can be placed anywhere – there is a plethora of places available. So they expect to be treated with courtesy and to have an experience – both in getting on to a course and then once on it – which is designed to be user-friendly, interesting and fun, as well as hard work and intellectually satisfying. Staff, in return, expect students to honour their commitments to work, to contribute and participate in the learning activities. Together this commitment may be expressed in a learning contract, signed up to by both parties. On both sides the attitude is that of adult to adult, each bringing their own unique life experiences to contribute to the learning process.

What are the other things that have also changed? Institutional bureaucracy – a necessary thing but something which occasionally seems to *drive* rather than *support* the institution – has undergone radical overhaul in many places to ensure that processes are easier without being less efficient. This has made admission policies and procedures more streamlined and easier. There is also greater coordination amongst departments and institutions, e.g. to facilitate the fairly frequent transfer of both students and their credit either from one department to another or from one institution to another.

The major shift in academic attitudes is huge, as many of you will bear witness if you have undertaken recent study in higher education, especially if your only previous experience of post-school education was your nursing or midwifery training. More of that later! One of the most marked changes has been in the role of teachers. They are there to facilitate learning and to make learning a positive and enjoyable experience, for which the student, importantly, has to take significant responsibility. Didactic direction is a thing of the past. Passive receipt of information is not something with which you should be involved as a lifelong learner.

Probably the biggest change, certainly within the field of lifelong learning, has been in the positive explosion of teaching and learning methods in the last 20 years. Distance learning, open learning and work-based learning are all available. You can use all types of media, at all times of the day and night, to suit your needs. Watch TV at 2 a.m. if that is the only time available to you; study from high-quality written materials at a time, place and pace to suit yourself; use floppy disks or CD-ROM to extend the usefulness of your computer (or someone else's). If you want to add some human interaction you can still do taught courses, which are likely to include project work, peer support, peer learning and networking – not to mention cooperation with industry and a variety of work-based placements. And if you are not familiar with all these terms and techniques, never fear. There are a range of good and interesting sources of information on the market to explain them in detail for you.

If you have not studied for a long time, there are a range of courses available to help you. Formal access courses, which are designed to prepare you for study and give you the necessary knowledge building blocks to ensure that you start a course with at least as good a chance as everyone else of being successful, are an excellent route back into formal learning. Such courses are usually designed for those who, for whatever reason, have had a bad or non-existent school experience and who now want to exploit their own potential. They are frequently designed to take place over an academic year and to lead straight on into a specific programme at the same institution. Alternatively, there are shorter study skills courses, which are designed to help you brush-up on rusty skills and to help you regain confidence in your ability to study, to reintroduce you to some old study skills and to introduce you to some new ones.

I hope that this brief look at the changes in education that have happened as a result of the lifelong learning movement has made you curious, at the very least, about the changes. More than that, I hope that it has made you eager to experience some of these changes for yourself – I am sure that you will not be disappointed. If you are already a fan of lifelong learning, then you will need no further persuading. You only have to worry about what you are going to do next. Let us now move on to look at some of the changes in the world of work which have, at least in part, both driven and responded to the changes in education. We will then consider the idea of continuing professional development and explore that in more detail.

But first, to the world of work.

THE WORLD OF WORK

Education, of course, does not – or should not – exist in a vacuum. Education, amongst its many other functions, prepares people for work and offers new skills for those already working. Once again, the debate is not new – it is a debate that was already taking place in 1970s. Edgar Schein, an organization and career development specialist writing in the 1970s, articulated how the needs of an organization and the individual are (or should be) interdependent and that, in developing and managing careers, their aims are to match respective needs so that both benefit. He identified those needs as (Schein 1978):

- the organization's need to recruit, manage and develop human resources in order to maintain its effectiveness, survive and grow
- the individual's need to find work situations which provide security, challenges and opportunities for self-development throughout an entire life cycle.

Roger Dale (1985) remarked that: 'it [is] almost commonplace that the education history of the past 150 years or so has been marked by continuing attempts to link the education system more closely to the economy, to make schools solve the needs of industry more effectively'. Sir Bryan Nicholson, Chairman of the CBI Task Force on Training introduces *Towards a Skills Revolution: a Youth Charter* (Vocational Education and Training Task Force 1989) with the words: 'the debate on education and training has often been concerned with structures and delivery and too little concerned with outcomes'. Every year as the A level and Higher results are announced, there is a growing clamour from industry that, despite the fact that the results continue to improve, the core skills of literacy, numeracy, communication and IT remain below those required by the world of work.

Remind yourself again of the objectives of the Dearing report on the purposes of higher education cited earlier in this chapter. I make no apology for repeating them again here – they are of such importance. Three of the four objectives have a reference to the relevance of work (my emphases):

- to inspire and enable individuals to develop their capabilities to the highest potential throughout life, so that they grow intellectually, *are well equipped for work*, can contribute effectively to society and achieve personal fulfilment
- to increase knowledge and understanding for their own sake and to foster their application *to the benefit of the economy* and society
- to *serve the needs of an adaptable, sustainable, knowledge based economy* at local, regional and national levels.

Charles Handy, my own personal guru, has been telling us for many years that the way we organize our work and careers will need major refashioning and overhaul if we are going to cope with the changes demanded by the world of work (Handy 1989, 1991, 1994, 1995). Writing in 1995 he comments on how much has changed in the last 10 years. The main change has been away from the certainty of the Thatcher and Reagan years (right or wrong though they may have been) to the confusion of the post-communist world and renewed conflict in places like the former Yugoslavia. Certainty went out – experiment came in with a vengeance.

Whilst working in Yugoslavia in 1996, I had the privilege of meeting a young doctor, who acted as my translator, who was saying how desperately difficult it is to bring up children in a world where all your previous values and beliefs had been overturned and not replaced. 'What do you say to children about their future,' she said, 'when there is so much uncertainty. At least before we knew that if we worked hard and studied we could be sure of a good job that was well paid and a secure future. Now all that counts for nothing'. She had been paid 2000 Deutschmarks (DM) a month before the recent Balkans war, 5 DM a month during the war and 400 DM afterwards. She had just given up medicine to work for a drug company, as she could no longer afford to feed her growing family. But far more important to her was what values and belief systems she and her husband should now seek to instil into their children.

Let us return to Charles Handy for a while and his vision of the new world of life and work. Handy describes four 'ages' in human lives (Handy 1995):

- The *first age* is that age in which we prepare for life and work. This includes both schooling and preparation for careers and the world of work. It is also the age in which we 'form' ourselves (from the French *formation*) in terms of values and beliefs, through our experiences at home and beyond.
- The *second age* is that of our 'main endeavours'. This may be through a variety of activity, e.g. paid work, rearing a family, creating works of art.
- The *third age* is the one which would come as a surprise to our grandparents – and indeed to many from other cultures today. This is the time for a second life. It might be a continuation of the first but it is just as likely, and very interestingly, to be something significantly different.
- The *fourth age*, which hopefully is as short as possible, is the age of dependency.

Handy also describes four types of 'work', which are not synonymous with the four ages: *paid* work, for which we receive wages or fees; *gift* work which we do for free – for the community or a charity or a sports club; *home* work, which includes child-rearing and the care of dependants, not to mention the catering, laundry, transport, gardening, decorating services that are included; and *study* work, which is the subject of this book. He describes the latter as 'an essential investment' and the acquisition and development of intelligence, knowledge and skill as 'the new form of property'.

How and why has Handy identified these issues and what is their relevance to us? He describes 'a vast reconfiguration of the world of work' which is happening right before our eyes. Heightened competition in the global market place is, he believes, driving this radical change. Office buildings are emptying as organizations shed their workforces and reconfigure the nature of employment. Only those who manage the 'core' business will have a permanent contract. Far more people will be used in a different way, e.g. as consultants, pieceworkers or temporary workers of some kind, people who will be brought in when there is work to be done but who are 'released' when that piece of work is completed, until the next occasion when there is something for them to do. He originally described the new 'shape' of work as a shamrock, but more recently as a three-ringed circle. The inner circle consists of the 'corporate insiders' – the entrepreneurs, the highly trained executives, the technicians and the salespersons. The outer ring consists of the 'interchangeable and disposable' – those who are pulled in and out of work according to demand. This tends to be the less skilled workforce and is certainly not a new phenomenon. What is new is the middle ring. This is where you increasingly find what Handy calls the 'portfolio' people – those people who do not intend to spend a lifetime with a particular organization, even if that were an option. They have a portfolio of marketable skills which can be used in a variety of settings. They have a product, skill or service which has a market and they sell their skills within that market.

Portfolio people, Handy says, may not have adopted that lifestyle willingly; it may have been forced upon them or they may have embraced it with enthusiasm and choice. Either way, you can soon see what it leads to. The notion of work as a straight line – school → qualification → first job → experience → promotion → more experience and promotion – until it stops dead at retirement (that isn't meant to be taken too literally, although regrettably it often proves to be the case) will soon be a thing of the past, if it is not already. Portfolio careers will be more circular, their rewards becoming more variable – some in kind, some in money, some in freedom to organize your own time, increased personal satisfaction in doing a range of things. How does it sound, terrifying or invigorating? Personally I think it sounds wonderful! More of that a bit later.

I hope this is all starting to come together. If you put the four ages and the four types of work together with the changing face of work, you will see the changing picture that Handy is building up. The types of work and the ages become increasingly blurred. If you are in the inner ring of the pattern, the chances are that you will be working at least 70-80 hours a week, totally committed to your workplace and having little time or energy to do other things, whether that be having children, taking holidays, engaging in anything outside work. There is nothing wrong with this lifestyle if you like it, but it will not last. People run the risk of becoming burnt out, exhausted and low on creativity. How about a time of portfolio working? Have a change – spread your skills; refocus your life; work out what is really important to you; mix and match your 'types' of work; change the proportion of time spent in each area. Re-enter the inner circle in due course if you want to.

Personally, I think this all sounds great and am currently realizing my own personal ambition to have my own portfolio career. Having spent the last 12 years working in London, commuting 120 miles each day by car, train and tube, leaving home in the morning at 6.20 and rarely returning before 7.30 in the evening, I decided that I wanted a change. I had loved what I was doing, but didn't want to go on with that lifestyle indefinitely. I now work from home, with my computer as my umbilical cord to the world. I sit in my study in rural Hampshire, looking out on to Watership Down, receiving e-mails, faxes and phone calls, and even occasionally something by snail mail (with apologies to the postman) from friends and colleagues all over the world. I undertake consultancies for a variety of organizations, including the World Health Organization and the International Council of Nurses, I write a lot, both articles and books, I do speaking engagements on a variety of subjects and undertake a range of other work as it comes my way. It's wonderful. *And*, best of all, I have time for a life outside work! I may not do it indefinitely. Who knows, at some stage I may choose to enter 'the inner circle' again – that will depend on a whole range of things, but this is an experience I would not have missed for the world.

Of course, such a Utopia provides its own challenges. Lots of things need to change to accommodate these changes: more portable pension schemes; more use of technology; 24 hour access to a range of services, like banking, shopping, and so on. But these things are happening, aren't they? Just look around you and see what is available. Shops are open on Sundays and until late, food and goods can be bought by computer. Banking is available by phone 24 hours a day. How long will it be before we are able to have our cars serviced overnight or, miracle of miracles, an appointment to see your own GP before 8 a.m. or after 8 p.m.? There is already a drop-in health clinic on Liverpool Street station in London, staffed by nurses and doctors and open all day and evening.

Look at some of the other changes that are happening in the world of work. Part-time hours are being used more imaginatively, and there is a significant increase in the number of jobs being advertised where there is a possibility of a job-share, the employer thus gaining the skills and knowledge of two people rather than one. There is the possibility of increasingly interesting part-time work, weekend work, annual hours contracts, zero hours contracts (being available for work only when it is available), paternity leave, career breaks and sabbaticals – just to give you a flavour of what is available. The other change that will happen in the 'new' world of work is that people will no longer expect that any change will always be onwards and upwards. There will be more horizontal movement as individuals move across structures for more experience and renewed interest. Organization structures are getting noticeably flatter, as hierarchies lose their relevance in the era of the individual who is employed for what they bring to the job, not merely for the number of years that they have served.

People are increasingly becoming encouraged to work from home, at least for part of their working week, if their work is of the type where at least some of it can be done in any setting. This reduces the amount of office space needed and also puts the time spent travelling into more productive use. Office space diminishes with open planning, hot-desking (used by whoever happens to be in the office that day) and the use of a lap-top for mobility and a fax with your PC at home. E-mail means that there is now a cheap and efficient way of being in contact with distant parts of the world for the cost of a local phone call. The Internet gives you access to information beyond the wildest expectations of more traditional information sources. The world can literally be at your fingertips.

Just in case you think I am writing about a world that does not concern you, stop and reflect for a while on some of the changes you have witnessed recently, even if you were not aware at the time that they were manifestations of a veritable revolution. At what time of day/night can you now go shopping? When did you last actually need to go into a bank? How many people do you know who have been made redundant or have taken early retirement because there has been a 'downsizing' of the workforce? How many more people are now employed on a contractual basis, whether as a consultant or agency or bank staff? Who amongst your friends has an open-ended contract; how many more are on fixed term ones?

In an article in *The Guardian* in 1997 (24 September), John Vidal offers the following proposed schedule as a way in which what he calls 'the 24 hour society' may develop in the future:

1 a.m.	Go swimming, increasing pressures on institutions to adapt to new life styles.
2 a.m.	Visit doctor and pharmacy. Check bank account, pay bills.
4.30 a.m.	Work for the Thai group selling hotel space. More jobs are being created, many global.
8.30 a.m.	Sleep. We still need it but may have to get used to ignoring the night.
4.30 p.m.	Drop children at school. Everyone may now have to adapt to new time pressures.
5 p.m.	Work for German research firm. People have different jobs, many of which they will do in their 'own' time.
9 p.m.	Take car for servicing. The night economy is booming.
10 p.m.	Pick up children. Watch television.
11.30 p.m.	Eat in restaurant, visit pub. Everything is open all the time.
12.30 a.m.	Visit stress counsellor. With everything open all the time, life is more rushed than ever.

Well, what do you think – exciting, nerve-racking, totally off the wall? Let's wait and see.

In relation to the way that our work is organized, we only have to look at the changes in the delivery of the health services since the turn of the decade and think of the effects – personal and professional – that the changes have had, and will have, on numerous employees: the imposition of the internal market, the purchaser/provider split, directly managed units, the establishment of trusts, commissioning, fund-holding GP practices, the merging of trusts, the demise of the internal market, the creation of health action zones, GP commissioning pilot projects, private finance initiatives. The list appears endless. I'm not raising the issues to comment on whether the reforms have been good or bad – they are probably rather like the curate's egg, good in parts – but merely to indicate the speed and ferocity of the changes and the huge impact they have had on the way we work.

We have not yet touched on the nature of the knowledge needed to cope with the demands of these changes. Depending on whose estimates you use, the amount of knowledge needed for most forms of work will change significantly every 4–7 years and this time-span is dropping all the time. This poses enormous challenges to those currently working, and even greater challenges to the group that we have not even started to address yet – those who are out of work for any reason. And this is where the relevance of this

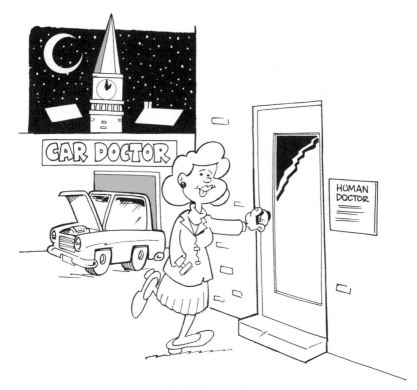

The 24-hour society.

discussion becomes clear. The implications of these changes will have a huge impact on the need for lifelong learning, and indeed will have been the driver for the changes in lifelong learning in many instances.

How does all this impact on the subject of this chapter? Hugely, of course. If we are to accept that the nature and pattern of work is going to – or indeed already is – changing so significantly, then the implications and opportunities for lifelong learning are almost unlimited. The changing nature of work over our lifetimes will require a whole new approach to the acquisition of knowledge and skills. No-one can or should feel complacent that the knowledge and skills acquired at the point of qualification remain relevant to meet all the changes of the modern world of work.

That bald statement needs some unpicking right away, though, or the book will lose a large percentage of its readership right now! At least, I hope that a number of you reading this fall into the category of being currently out of practice but thinking of coming back to nursing, midwifery or health visiting at some stage in the near future. And given that one of the reasons for the book is to encourage people to return to work without being terrified of all the changes, I don't want to dwell too much on the nature of change without offering some positive, workable solutions for managing people's concerns.

One of the biggest concerns people have, and something that often paralyses them in the face of change, is the fear that they will not be able to cope with what that change involves. I think this fear is reasonable and understandable but I do not accept that it is a valid excuse for refusing to try something different. Who knows, you may love the difference!

It is worth looking in more detail at what causes that fear. It might be a generalized fear of the unknown. It might be fear of looking silly in front of others. It might be fear of actually doing something wrong and hurting someone or damaging expensive equipment. It may be a lack of knowledge. It is very likely to be a lack of confidence. These are all perfectly understandable and indeed commendable. Nothing is more dangerous than the person who is inappropriately confident but inexperienced. We only have to look at the accident statistics for young drivers to get the evidence for that. So, where does the answer lie? I believe it lies in effective, well planned, relevant, continuing professional development. You thought I might just say that, didn't you?

Let's look at what that actually means.

CONTINUING PROFESSIONAL DEVELOPMENT

Continuing professional development is the term given to the learning which takes place in a professional's career after the point of qualification and/or registration. It can be considered within the broad area of lifelong learning and will have many of the characteristics identified earlier in this chapter. Most importantly, perhaps, is that CPD is identified and intentional learning – this is not the term for the learning which comes from the experience of professional practice.

According to Madden & Mitchell (1993), who undertook a substantial survey of the professions in the early 1990s, continuing professional development has become 'the term widely used for continuing education in all the professions'. They go on to say that it is a distinctive part of continuing vocational education, which has been one of the major growth areas in the last 15 years. The definition they use of continuing professional development is:

the maintenance of and enhancement of knowledge, expertise and competence of professionals throughout their careers according to a plan formulated with regard to the needs of the professional, the employer, the profession and society.

More importantly, they offer a definition of *effective* CPD which is relevant to our topic in hand, as follows: 'the aim of effective CPD is to provide a profession whose members are fully trained and competent to perform the tasks expected of them throughout their careers'. This is a useful definition and would, I believe, gain a lot of favour with those with an interest in this area of education and practice. And who are they? At first sight, they seem to form a surprisingly wide group, although when you come to think about it, all those named do have a legitimate interest in the subject.

The largest group with an interest is, of course, *society* (if, that is, you believe there is such a thing!). Individual members of society are the ones who are going to be at the receiving end of the knowledge and skills of the professionals in the particular profession with whom they are interacting at any one time. They (we!) have a right to expect those who profess to a certain body of knowledge and skills to be able to deliver their 'goods', whether that be, for example, sound legal advice, knowledgeable and compassionate nursing care, effective medicine, or well prepared and accurate teaching.

Employers also have – or should have – an overriding interest in CPD. It must be in the interests of a good employer to have staff who are both initially well qualified and who then take every effort to maintain and develop their profession-specific knowledge and competence. Given the speed of change of both knowledge and skills in most professions, ensuring that your workforce, to be blunt, knows what it is doing, is vital. An increasingly knowledgeable and litigious public both expect and demand competence in those to whom they pay their money, whether as a direct fee or an indirect taxation.

The *government* also has a legitimate interest in CPD. Not least because, ultimately, any central support for training – of which there is a considerable amount, even if it doesn't seem immediately apparent to those on the ground – costs money, which is frequently found, at least in some part, from the public coffers, by one route or another. In addition, as the role of the professions comes under increasing scrutiny, in all areas, particularly the self-regulating professions, there are those in a variety of fields who feel that the professions have had the monopoly on power and influence for too long and cannot continue to rest on their laurels without increasingly visible lines of accountability. Explicit CPD requirements contribute to that visibility and accountability.

The *statutory bodies and professional bodies*, depending on the exact terms of their roles and functions, will also have considerable interest in the CPD issue – indeed a central role in many instances. This issue is worth expanding at this stage, as there is a lot of confusion about role and function. Statutory regulatory bodies are set up by legislation with a specific remit, which they are required by their enabling legislation – the Act of Parliament (the primary legislation) – to fulfil. That remit will usually relate broadly, and to a greater or lesser extent, to standards of education/training, conduct/discipline and registration. Their prime purpose is the protection of the public and it is, or should be, to this end that all their activities are targeted. The statutory regulatory bodies in the health field are the United Kingdom Central Council for Nursing, Midwifery and Health Visiting, the General Medical Council, the General Dental Council, the Royal Pharmaceutical Society of Great Britain, the General Optical Council and the (current but under review) Council for the Professions Supplementary to Medicine.

Then there are the professional bodies, who may also have a trade union function. Professional bodies, such as the Royal College of Nursing or the Royal College of Midwives, are often set up under Royal Charter and their function relates to the furtherance of the profession concerned, through professional practice and education. They will frequently provide a range of guidance and literature in the area of professional practice. Some professional bodies will have the responsibility for standards of professional practice beyond registration. In some professions, membership of the relevant professional body is essential for practice of that profession and the practitioner must meet whatever requirements are in place for membership, which may include CPD requirements.

The exact detail of the range of responsibilities in a particular profession will vary between the statutory and professional bodies. For example, the UKCC is required to set standards for pre- and post-registration education. The four National Boards for nursing, midwifery and health visiting have the power to approve the institutions who offer the programmes of education. The General Medical Council, on the other hand, has responsibility for pre-registration education. It is the medical royal colleges which have responsibility for post-registration education. As the functions can be different in significant ways, interested individuals should always check or confusion may result.

The *individual practitioner* has a considerable interest in their own profession's CPD requirements. The first thing that they need, of course, is accurate knowledge. First things first. Are there CPD requirements in place? If there are, are they statutory, mandatory or permissive? When do they start? How often do they have to be met? Who sets the standards? What are the sanctions for non-compliance? What are the options for meeting the requirements? Let us look at this in some more detail.

Statutory, mandatory or permissive?

What is the difference between these terms? They are frequently used inaccurately but that is unnecessary if you look at the origins of the words.

Statutory. As the word suggests its origins will be found in statute or legislation, being required, permitted or enacted by statute. To put it simply you *have* to do it because it is the law. Make sure you have the spelling right and don't muddle it up with carving marble and the like, which is known as statuary! I suppose that things could get confusing if you have a statute enacted from an ivory tower – or am I being too clever for my own good? The PREP requirements are statutory and are set out in a *statutory instrument* or *rule* (Ch. 5 has more details)

Mandatory. This term is frequently used when the user really means statutory. A mandate is an official command or instruction by an authority.

Mandatory, in practice, means compulsory. Some CPD requirements will be mandatory for membership of that particular profession, e.g. the chartered accountants, although they are not actually set out in law. In practice, as far as the individual is concerned, this may be a purely semantic difference.

Permissive. Here, the individual has a choice. The approach is liberal and tolerant – take it or leave it, do it or don't do it. On the face of it, not very powerful, but with peer pressure, it can be quite effective. The difficulty, however, comes with the type of sanctions which can be imposed if an individual chooses to exercise their authority not to do something and is then found to be wanting in some area of their practice.

What type of CPD?

In their survey of continuing education for the professions, Madden & Mitchell (1993) identified two broad models of provision of CPD. They referred to them as the 'sanctions' and 'benefits' models. The *sanctions* model is the one which tends to be used most by the highly visible and well established professions, who have powerful, professional or regulatory bodies. Such an approach goes with a model of fairly firm professional control, where entry, length, exit, registration, standards and discipline are explicit and formally and firmly policed. If there is no compliance with the required standards, then sanctions of some type will come into play. Such an approach is adopted by, amongst others, the Law Society, the Institute of Chartered Accountants in England and Wales, and the Royal Institute of British Architects.

The *benefits* model has a significantly different approach. CPD is introduced to assure the continued and enhanced competence of the members of the profession in question and may lead to academic- or competency-based qualifications. The emphasis is on the outcomes of CPD for practice and is linked to the notion of reward for undertaking CPD, rather than sanctions for non-compliance. The results are implicit rather than explicit, and taking part in CPD becomes 'the thing to do' and is looked for by employers as active evidence of commitment to the profession. The Central Council for the Education and Training of Social Workers (CETSW) adopt this approach, as do the Institute of Personnel Managers. One does not have to be a member of IPM for employment, and therefore compliance with their CPD scheme cannot be a prerequisite for practice. On the other hand, it is considered by the profession and employers alike as evidence of professional commitment (Peel 1995).

Such a model is of interest, although it does not provide the whole answer for CPD schemes within the professions. Some systems are a mixture of both models or are moving from one approach to another. This is discussed in more detail in the next chapter, looking at approaches to professional regulation.

The system in question

All professionals should be aware of what CPD requirements are in place in their own particular profession. The only reason that it is an issue for nurses and health visitors is because such requirements are comparatively new. Within a very short space of time, all newly qualified registrants will know that continuing education in the form of the PREP requirements is just part and parcel of being registered. Ask any midwife. Midwives have had the benefit of statutory requirements for continuing education since the 1930s. All midwives are made aware of the legislative requirements which are currently set out in Rule 37 of the Midwives Rules (UKCC 1993) during their training, in relation to refresher courses, so they enter professional practice – and have done so within the memory of every practising midwife – in the full knowledge of what is expected of them.

To take another example from a profession with which many of you will be familiar – teaching (with apologies to Scotland and Northern Ireland for the English and Welsh example).The 1989 Education Act in England and Wales introduced the notion of what are colloquially known as 'Baker days' (or INSET days, in-service education and training) for the teaching profession. You have probably been at the receiving end of their implementation. They are the days that your children come home and tell you about, just after the off-duty has been done for the next month! 'Mum/Dad, I've got the day off next Monday 'cos the teachers are doing a course on managing neglected children.' You know the sort of thing. When I asked my husband – who's a headteacher – about the requirements, he said that they have already become 'part of the fabric of things'. To have entered the professional consciousness in that way within 7 years is pretty good going, I think. My daughter and son-in-law, who have both entered teaching within the last 3 years, accept INSET days as part and parcel of their professional practice. There is no formal approval of INSET activity and it is decided on a school-by-school basis to meet the needs of the organization as well as the individual teachers. Much of the activity takes place within the schools themselves, although sometimes external speakers are brought in or a course is undertaken externally. The costs are borne by the school as part of their INSET budget.

Who sets the standards?

It never fails to amaze me how accepting some people are of some of the things that are imposed upon them, without wanting to know who it is that has set the requirements and why. If there are standards in place that affect me, I want to know who has said what, where, why, is it optional, mandatory or statutory and what are the routes for challenge. Many people seem to be quite content to blame the ubiquitous 'they' for a lot of things, without anyone bothering to find out who 'they' are. Numerous practitioner phone calls to the UKCC's helpline to ask about something that is causing the individual and/or their colleagues concern go something like this:

'I/we have got a problem with X, which we have been told we have to do.'
'Who says you have to do it?'
'It's the policy.'
'Whose policy?'
'Well, I'm not sure. *They* say we have to do it.'
'Who are they – the Trust, your immediate boss, the National Board? '
'We thought it was the UKCC.'
'No, this is not something on which the UKCC has issued a policy.'
'Well, I don't know then....'
'Perhaps it would be worth finding out before we go any further...'

and so on and so on.

So, the moral is, find out whose CPD standards you have to meet. For nurses, midwives and health visitors it is the PREP requirements, set by the UKCC – just in case, you haven't already got that message! For other professions, it might be those of the statutory regulatory body concerned, or the relevant professional organization or the Royal College. Your employer may also have set additional standards which are part of your contractual responsibilities. Make sure that you know who has said and set what.

Sanctions

It is extremely important for the professionals concerned to be quite clear about the CPD arrangements in their own particular profession, particularly the sanctions that will be imposed for non-compliance. This becomes a matter of particular significance where there is a risk of losing one's registration – and therefore the right to practise – if the requirements are not met. It is important to know what the sanctions are and whether there are any circumstances in which a dispensation can be made for non-compliance. Most importantly, how does one get one's registration back if one is unfortunate enough to lose it? What are the mechanisms and costs?

The usefulness of CPD

The Institute of Management (Peel 1995) described CPD as an 'attitude of mind rather than a mechanism'. They go on to say that CPD guidance used today is unlikely to have relevance in the short term – it may be years before practitioners can be motivated. Diane Turnbull and Margaret Holt of the University of Georgia (Turnbull & Holt 1993) in their consideration of a conceptual framework for evaluating continuing education in allied health concluded that 'the question of whether those who participate in continuing education practise with improved knowledge and skills or continue unchanged has not been rigorously researched'. When it has, they continued, the results are inconsistent. In their review, they evaluated 22 studies of continuing education in allied health and found that 17 evaluated only one outcome. One study only, that conducted by Woog & Hyman (1980), looked at satisfaction, knowledge, and application of knowledge after the programme. Even here, the results were mixed. Richardson (1981) attempted to look at any type of correlation between satisfaction, knowledge and application of learning after the programme. Although most of the allied health care literature in the United States has concentrated on the assessment of knowledge, other factors, such as satisfaction, impact on performance and, most importantly, impact on patient care have 'been largely ignored'. The article concluded that 'further research is needed in allied health to document the link between participation, satisfaction, knowledge and improvement in performance in the workplace'.

On this side of the Atlantic, much of the literature concentrates on process not outcome, particularly in the work done on nursing and midwifery. Very little systematic evaluation has been done of midwives' refresher courses in relation to the effect on the care given to mothers and babies. Lathlean (1986), when talking about continuing education schemes, recommends that:

emphasis in continuing education for all staff should be on systematic role-based development and on the provision of educational opportunities which are sufficiently flexible to accommodate differences between individuals and between different service requirements.

Nothing there about evaluation. Hughes (1990) tried to adopt a systematic approach to evaluating the impact of CPD. In her literature review she found that the evaluation of CPD activities is frequently limited to the completion of forms at the conclusion of the activity, indicating the extent to which the objectives had been achieved and the general level of satisfaction on the part of the participants. Very little attention was given to the longer term effects of CPD on either the individual participant or their ability to provide an enhanced level of nursing care. This finding was mirrored by Ferguson (1994) who identified that 'learner satisfaction or knowledge acquisition...are most usually evaluated'. There is an assumption that as knowledge, communication and assertiveness skills are increased, there is professional and educational development and the nurse's ability to improve patient care is enhanced (see review by Nolan et al 1995).

Nolan et al (1995), in their excellent paper, seek to identify the characteristics of an effective continuing professional education system. They comment that whilst the literature describes a number of benefits, detailed empirical studies have been limited. There is, in particular, a dearth of information on nurses' perceptions of the important components of CPE activity. Using a Donabedian structure, process and outcome model, attention is focused on the outcomes of CPE and those issues which impede or enhance success. Factors which inhibit success include (see review by Nolan et al 1995):

- time, money
- availability of good opportunities
- poor information/awareness
- workplace/workload pressures
- family commitments
- lack of encouragement from managers.

Staff selection for CPE activity is found to be 'arbitrary, random and inequitable' (Larcombe & Maggs 1991).

Benefits, however, can accrue and are identified in the same study (Nolan et al 1995) as better care planning (Hughes 1990), informal exchange of ideas between participants, greater assertiveness and autonomy (Hughes 1990), and staff becoming more competent and accountable. Sunter (1993) sums up the position very clearly: 'continuing education will survive and prosper in the market place if it is seen to be the "fittest"' for its purpose – the delivery of cost-effective quality care demonstrated through the enhanced performance of the professional'. All of us involved with CPD will have to take up this challenge and help to provide the evidence.

CONCLUSION

This chapter has tried to pull together issues relating to three major strands – those of lifelong learning, changes in the ways society's work is being organized and continuing professional development. It has looked at these changes from the perspective of our quest to put the work of PREP into context. Let us move on now to start to look at issues which are more specific to nursing, midwifery and health visiting.

REFERENCES

Ball C 1991 Learning pays. RSA, London
Barnett R 1990 The idea of higher education. SHRE and Open University Press, Buckingham
Barnett R 1992 Improving higher education. SHRE and Open University Press, Buckingham
Dale R 1985 Education, training and employment, towards a new vocationalism. Pergamon, London
Faure E 1972 Learning to be: the world of education today and tomorrow. UNESCO and Harrap Press, Paris
Ferguson A 1994 Evaluating the purpose and benefits of continuing education in nursing and the implications of the provision of continuing education for cancer nursing. Journal of Advanced Nursing 19(4): 640–645
Handy C 1989 The age of unreason. Hutchinson, London
Handy C 1991 Waiting for the mountain to move. Hutchinson, London
Handy C 1994 The empty raincoat. Hutchinson, London
Handy C 1995 Beyond certainty. Hutchinson, London
Hazlegrove S (ed) 1994 The student experience. SHRE and Open University Press, Buckingham
Hughes P 1990 The impact of continuing professional education. Nurse Education Today 10: 428–435

Knapper C, Croxley A 1985 Lifelong learning in higher education. Kogan Page, London

Larcombe K, Maggs C 1991 Processes for identifying the CPE needs of nurses, midwives and health visitors: an evaluation report for the English National Board for Nursing, Midwifery and Health Visiting, Project Paper 5. ENB, London

Lathlean J 1986 The ward sister training project, neighbourhood nursing. NERU, Kings College, London

Lawton D 1992 Education and politics in the 1990s – conflict or consensus, The Falmer Press, London

Lewis RG, Smith DH 1994 Total quality in higher education – continuous development. St Lucie Press, Florida

Madden CA, Mitchell VA 1993 Professional standards and competence. a survey of continuing professional education for the professions. University of Bristol, Department of Continuing Education, Bristol

National Committee of Inquiry into Higher Education 1997 Higher education in the learning society (Dearing report). HMSO, London

National Committee of Inquiry into Higher Education 1997 Higher education in a learning society – report of the Scottish Committee (Garrick report). HMSO, Norwich

Nolan M, Nolan J, Owens RG 1995 Continuing professional education: identifying the characteristics of an effective system. Journal of Advanced Nursing 21(3)

Peel M 1995 Develop or die. Institute of Management Conference on the Changing Role of Professional Associations, London

Pucheu R 1974 La formation permentante: idée neuvée? Idée fausse? Esprit 10: 321-336

Richardson G E 1981 A sexual health workshop for health care professionals. Evaluating Health Professionals 4: 259–274

Ruegg W 1974 Le role de l'université dans l'education permanente. CRE – Information 25: 3–20

Schein EH 1978 Career dynamics: matching individual and organizational needs. Addison Wesley, New York

Sunter S 1993 The effectiveness of continuing education. Nursing Standard 8(6): 37–39

Turnbull DC, Holt ME 1993 Conceptual frameworks for evaluating continuing education in allied health. Journal of Continuing Education in the Health Professions 13(2)

UKCC 1993 Midwives rules. UKCC, London

Vocational Education and Training Task Force 1991 Towards a skills revolution. Confederation of British Industry, London

Woog P, Hyman RB 1980 Evaluating continuing education: a focus on the client. Evaluating Health Professionals 3: 171–190

Vidal J 1997 *The Guardian*. 24 September, p 3

3

The changing face of professional regulation

Change is constant.

(*The Times*, Benjamin Disraeli)

INTRODUCTION

The previous chapter looked at the general issues surrounding lifelong learning, the changing face of work and continuing professional development, in order to provide a broad contextual backdrop for an exploration of specific initiatives within the nursing and midwifery professions. Before this exploration of context is complete and we turn to an explicit consideration of the PREP project, it is essential to examine briefly the whole concept of professional regulation, first from the point of principle and then, more specifically, how it is applied in the UK. Such an exploration is necessary in order to make sense of the subsequent work on PREP, in terms of how the project was conceived, nurtured and put into effect.

This chapter, therefore, looks first at the principles associated with professional regulation and examines how these principles are put into effect in the UK. It then moves from the systems to the individuals who put those systems into effect and explores the personal implications of a good regulation system for those whom it regulates. The concept of accountability is given particular attention. This exploration then provides the backdrop for a consideration of the work done by the UKCC during the 1980s and early 1990s, particularly in relation to the development of the Council's *Code of Professional Conduct* and the *Scope of Professional Practice* (UKCC 1992a,b). Together, these will provide the setting for consideration of the PREP project itself. Time, space and balance necessitate only a brief consideration of each of these important issues, each of which could (and, indeed, in many instances do) fill books on their own. However, I hope that they will at least be helpful in terms of context and also that they may arouse your interest sufficiently to explore the issues further, in due course.

PROFESSIONAL REGULATION

Few of us, I suspect, particularly if we have only had experience of professional regulation in the UK, realize how privileged we are. This is not in any way imperialist complacency speaking – I am not saying that the system that we have is the best, or indeed the only, model. But we do have an effective way of regulating the profession, which many other countries envy. In essence, the UK has the advantage of a system whereby the professionals concerned – nurses, midwives and health visitors – set their own standards of practice, education and conduct. 'But, of course,' you may say, if you have known no different. However, there are many countries where standards for nursing and midwifery are set, or significantly influenced, by others – be they lawyers, politicians, doctors, educationalists or civil servants. The nurses and midwives themselves have very little influence, if any, on their educational or practice standards, although many of them are fighting vigorously to bring about change. In contrast, there is a shamefully small percentage of the

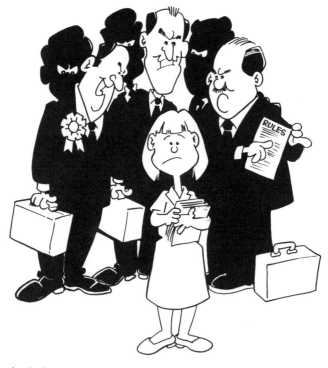

'... standards for nursing and midwifery are set, or significantly influenced, by others, whether it be lawyers, politicians, doctors, educationalists or civil servants.'

640 000 practitioners on the Council's register who vote in the UKCC elections (only 13% in the 1997 elections). Yet they are being asked to vote for those who will be responsible for setting the standards for nursing, midwifery and health visiting practice, education and conduct in the next 5 years and beyond. It is difficult not to conclude that the majority of those on the UKCC register do not really understand or value the system that we have in the UK.

Professional regulation – in its broadest, most principled sense – *matters*. Not the petty and rigid imposition of ancient rules and regulations, but the dynamic and vibrant vision of positively regulating the profession in the public interest, in a positive and supportive manner. It matters to the individual professional. It matters to the vulnerable public for whom we care. It matters to society. It matters to government. It matters to those who employ the nurses, midwives and health visitors.

The International Council of Nurses has undertaken some excellent work on the regulation of nursing (ICN 1985, Affara & Styles 1992), which was reviewed in 1996 (Pyne 1997) and which is applicable to midwifery and indeed many other professions. It would be helpful to look at this in some more detail here, so that we can put the UK activity within a broader framework. Regulation is defined as 'the forms and processes whereby order, consistency and control are brought to an occupation and its practice' (ICN 1985). In one sense, this does sound rather mechanistic, but when you go on to explore the principles that enhance the definition, it becomes clear that it is anything but mechanistic. Another strong proponent of regulation, Reg Pyne, professional conduct/standards and ethics supremo at the UKCC for many years, and now a well-respected consultant on professional issues, particularly within the field of professional regulation, elaborates further: 'regulation is also a substantial part of the means by which an occupational group which espouses the worthy title "profession" demonstrates and honours its accountability to the public and its associated commitment to serve the public interest' (Pyne 1997, unpublished work). He goes on to say: 'For the nursing/midwifery professions, as for any professions serving the public interest, an appropriate and effective system of professional regulation should not be seen as a distraction from professional practice, but an essential element of professional practice.'

What a good regulation system does is to ensure that relevant, responsive and effective standards are in place for the professionals whom it regulates. These standards need to be visible and arrived at after consultation with all those who will be affected by them. The standards can then serve a benchmark of quality for the public, the registrants themselves, other professions, the government and employers. This quality benchmark serves a number of useful purposes. It assures the public, employers and society at large that the nurse or midwife has acquired at least a minimum standard of knowledge and skill. It also makes it clear that such an individual can be called to account for inappropriate behaviour – whether that behaviour be due to misconduct or physical or mental ill-health. It also serves as a professional 'passport' for the individual should they want to move around the world. Other countries can then know what standards have been reached, in terms of professional education and practice.

Principles of professional regulation

In 1985, ICN published its report on the regulation of nursing. Before describing the 12 principles of regulation, the report concludes that 'the welfare of the public, the profession and the practitioner will be better served if greater relevance, consistency and clarity are brought to bear upon the regulatory system'. The report went on to describe 12 principles of professional regulation, as follows:

I   *Principle of purposefulness* – regulation should be directed towards a specific purpose

II   *Principle of relevance* – regulation should be designed to achieve its stated purpose

III *Principle of definition* – regulatory standards should be based on clear definitions of professional scope and accountability

IV   *Principle of professional ultimacy* – regulatory definitions should promote the fullest development of the profession commensurate with its potential social contribution

V   *Principle of multiple interests and responsibilities* – regulatory systems should recognize and properly incorporate the legitimate roles and responsibilities of interested parties – public, profession, government, employers, other professions – in aspects of standard-setting

VI   *Principle of representational balance* – the design of the regulatory system should acknowledge and appropriately balance interdependent interests

VII *Principle of optimacy* – regulatory systems should provide and be restricted to those controls and restrictions necessary to achieve their objectives

VIII *Principle of flexibility* – standards and processes of regulation should be sufficiently broad and flexible to achieve their objectives and at the same time permit freedom for innovation, growth and change

IX   *Principle of efficiency and congruence* – regulatory systems should operate in the most efficient manner, ensuring coherence and coordination among their parts

X   *Principle of universality* – regulatory systems should promote universal standards of performance and foster professional identity and mobility to the fullest extent compatible with local needs and circumstances

XI   *Principle of fairness* – regulatory processes should provide honest and just treatment for those parties regulated

XII   *Principle of interprofessional equality and compatibility* – in standards and processes regulatory system should recognise the equality and interdependence of professions.

In its fundamental review of its original report, the ICN reaffirmed these principles as relevant to practice into the millennium and beyond. They are of such importance as to warrant further exploration. I think it is important to look at each principle in turn and, given that the main focus of this book is the UK, to consider how effect is given to the principle under consideration by the UKCC. Thus, gradually we can fill in more of the contextual background against which the decisions on PREP were made and have a clearer view of why a particular approach was adopted, rather than another, on the issues under consideration.

The principle of purposefulness

Regulation should be directed towards a specific purpose. Regulation is about service to the public and public protection. It is about ensuring that all activity is focused on this aspect of its function. This involves ensuring that everything done in the name of regulation is directed towards its overarching goal. It means that the driver for any activity cannot be the good of the profession, but must be the greater protection of the potentially vulnerable public. Although there is appropriately increasing public involvement in the standards-setting work of the professions, on the whole, the public are still happy to leave this work to the professionals, confident that the standards set will be relevant. This position, however, may not continue, as the consumer rightly continues to exert authority where and when they feel they are not getting good value from the professions.

The UKCC has taken its responsibilities seriously in this regard. The systems set up to facilitate the work of the Council were, and continue to be, designed to keep public protection and safety in pole position. This applies not only to the obvious and frequently visible activity related to professional conduct, but also to its work on standards for education and practice. In practical terms, of course, one of the most important examples of public protection in action is the UKCC register. As one of the largest electronic data bases of its type in the world, let alone the UK, the register, with its thousands of changes each day, has to be meticulously managed, to ensure above all security and day-to-day accuracy of information

Principle of relevance

Regulation should be designed to achieve the stated purpose. The systems that are set up for any regulatory activity should be directed towards ensuring that they are relevant to the purpose of public protection. Standards for professional education and practice must meet these requirements. Does professional education produce a practitioner who is knowledgeable, skilled and competent? Are the educational standards subject to regular review to ensure that their relevance is maintained, within a rapidly changing context in relation to the organization and delivery of health care? Are standards set for practice, and if so, are they regularly reviewed? Are they really relevant to what happens in the clinical or practical situation or are they actually unachievable in reality? Who is responsible for maintaining the standards – is it the responsibility of the individual professional or are there other agencies? If so, what is their interest or angle? Does the practitioner work in a setting where it is possible to uphold appropriate standards? Who supports the individual if they are not convinced that the standards do meet the requirements for public safety? Who supports the individual practitioner in exercising their professional accountability, especially when there are differences of views?

Principle of definition

Regulatory standards should be based upon clear definitions of professional scope and accountability. This is an interesting point and one which has different approaches in different countries. In the UK, there are broad outcome statements in the training rules relating to the programmes leading to qualification as a nurse, midwife or health visitor. For example, Rule 18A(2) states first a stem and then 13 outcomes relating to aspects of nursing care, as follows (HMSO 1989):

Stem: 18A(2) The Common Foundation Programme and the Branch Programme shall be designed to prepare the student to assume the responsibilities and accountability that registration confers, and to prepare the nursing student to apply knowledge and skills to meet the nursing needs of individuals and of groups in health and in sickness in the area of the Branch Programme and shall include enabling the student to achieve the following outcomes: [*examples only given*]

(a) the identification of the social and health implications of pregnancy and child bearing, physical and mental handicap, disease, disability, or aging for the individual, his or her friends, family or community…
(e) an understanding of the requirements of legislation relevant to the practice of nursing….
(i) the identification of the needs of patients and clients to enable them to progress from varying degrees of dependence to maximum independence, or to a peaceful death.

There are no practice rules for nurses or health visitors, although there are for midwives. The midwives practice rules relate to matters such as notification of intention of practice, refresher course, suspension from practice, records, administration of medicines and responsibility and spheres of practice. The rules can be quite specific, as in Rule 41(3):

Unless special exemption is given by the Council to enable a particular hospital, or other institution, to investigate new methods, a practising midwife must not administrate any form of pain relief by the use of any type of apparatus or by any other means, which has not been approved by the Council other than on the instructions of a registered medical practitioner.

On the whole, though, they are more flexible in order to allow the individual practitioner to use their skill and judgement, as in Rule 40 which states:

A practising midwife is responsible for providing midwifery care to a mother and baby during the antenatal, intranatal and postnatal period. In any case where there is an emergency or where she detects in the health of a mother or baby a deviation from the norm, a practising midwife shall call to her assistance a registered medical practitioner and shall forthwith report the mother to the local supervising authority in a form in accordance with the requirements of the local supervising authority. (UKCC 1993)

This make it quite clear that the midwife is responsible for normal births, but should use her professional judgement as to when to call for assistance.

This contrasts with the legislation in some countries where the actual 'tasks' of nursing are laid down in legislation and the practitioner may *only* do that which is in the legislation. The more flexible approach adopted in the UK legislation means that the scope of professional practice can be very broad and this has facilitated the development of the UKCC document the *Scope of Professional Practice* (see p. 54).

Principle of professional ultimacy

Regulatory definitions and standards should promote the fullest development of the profession commensurate with its potential social contribution. This is a fundamental principle which goes right to the heart of regulation. It is asking the society and professions concerned to be quite clear about the profession's role within that society Where nursing and midwifery are valued, then the regulatory systems will reflect the accountability and scope of practice of those professionals. Where the professions are considered to be either unimportant or subsidiary to others, then either there will be no systems of regulation or they will be designed merely as an adjunct to others (almost invariably medicine).This is a complex and multifaceted issue, often linked with the role and perception of women in the particular society and the 'masculine' nature of decision-making, an issue fascinatingly explored by Celia Davies in her book *Gender and the Professional Predicament in Nursing* (Davies 1995).

It is an issue which is coming under considerable scrutiny in the UK as the debates become ever more focused on the nature of professional practice as well as exploring and challenging the traditional roles and boundaries between different professions. Nurses and midwives are not only taking on responsibilities previously associated with other professions, but also forging new roles for themselves. As consumer needs change over time, so nursing roles advance and expand, as nurses identify new approaches to their professional practice. The expansion in the role of mental health nursing, particularly in the community, is one good example of such changing practice. Midwives, too, have already been an integral part of such a movement in England with the *Changing Childbirth* initiative (Department of Health 1993). Such initiatives are welcomed by the public, who appear content to receive care from those who are demonstrably expert in their work, regardless of professional background.

Principle of multiple interests and responsibilities

Regulatory systems should recognise and properly incorporate the legitimate roles and responsibilities of interested parties – public, profession, government, employers, other professions – in aspects of standard setting and administration. Regulation is of interest to everyone. This is amply demonstrated by the public outcry through the vehicle of the press when one of the regulatory bodies – usually the General Medical Council or the UKCC – makes a professional conduct decision which does not appear to be commensurate with the offence under consideration.

The UKCC has worked increasingly hard during its lifetime to ensure that those with a legitimate interest in its business have a true and proper say in its affairs. Indeed, such a requirement is enshrined in the primary legislation, when new rules are to be made.

Section 19 of The Nurses, Midwives and Health Visitors Act 1997 requires that:

19(3) before making any rules under this Act, the Council shall consult –
(a) representatives of any group of persons who appear likely to be affected by the proposed rules; and
(b) the National Boards for the parts of the United Kingdom to which the proposed rules are to extend.

The wording of this section of the Act is significant – the Council *shall...*, i.e. it is a legal imperative, not an optional nicety. In other words, the Council *must* consult 'representatives of any group of person who appear likely to be affected by the proposed rules'. Again, here there is a wide-ranging requirement to be as inclusive as possible when consulting. Mere tokenism will not do. Were the Council not to exercise this responsibility in accordance with the law, then it could be called to account for its actions or omissions.

How does the Council choose who to consult? To an extent, this has to be a matter of judgement and will depend on the issue at hand. For example, when there was a request to change the term 'mental handicap' to 'learning disability' nursing, it had already become clear that this was a move which would receive widespread support. The organizations consulted, therefore, were those with direct links with this client group, being representatives

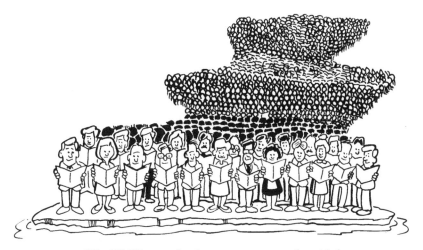

'The PREP consultation … was extremely wide.'

either of those working in the field or of those being cared for. The PREP consultation, on the other hand, came right at the other end of the consultation spectrum, as its proposals potentially affected every single practitioner on the register and many others, including employers: consultation was therefore extremely wide.

Let us return again to the wording of this important principle. Who has 'legitimate roles and responsibilities'? Although this is often self-evident, there can be actual or potential conflict when there is a divergence of opinion about the legitimacy of views. This is not necessarily an easy road to travel and calls for clear thinking, courage and clarity of purpose on behalf of the Council's members and officers.

One example concerned the response of the representatives of hospital consultants when they discovered (very late in the day, for some reason) that the UKCC was using the word 'specialist' for nurses. They were apparently concerned that patients might be confused and misled by those other than doctors calling themselves specialists. This required delicate untangling. Of course, it is important that patients are not misled and steps should always be taken to ensure that they are fully informed of who is looking after them and their relevant qualifications. However, one also has to be sure that this is not merely a touch of vested self-interest and inappropriate 'intervention' in the work of another profession. The term 'specialist' is, after all, used within a number of occupational groups.

There are also occasions on which the UKCC must, or should, take a stand against actual or proposed government policy, e.g. where that is not felt by the Council to be in the public interest. Again, this is not necessarily easy to do, and indeed there are those who feel that UKCC policy is increasingly and inappropriately influenced by government, potentially compromising its role as an independent body.

Principle of representational balance

The design of the regulatory system should acknowledge and appropriately balance interdependent interests. This is an interesting issue and one which will have different facets, depending on the organization of health care in the country concerned. In some countries, the regulatory body manages both the professionals and the support staff and will therefore have both groups represented on the governing body, in some form. Others, depending on their origins and the power and status of the professions of nursing and/or midwifery, will have heavy representation from other professions, such as medicine and the law, or from government.

In the UK, there are, again, different facets, representing both geographical and professional interests. These have been the subject of discussion and debate since the inception of the UKCC and four National Boards. There are the obvious geographical differences associated with the four countries of England, Scotland, Northern Ireland and Wales – an important issue which took on a whole new significance in 1997 with the devolution decisions for a Scottish Parliament and a Welsh Assembly. There is currently equal representation from all four countries – 10 members from each, seven nurses, two midwives and one health visitor. This is an issue which has been hotly debated by each successive Council, the professional organizations and the profession. There are those who argue that the current distribution of places is grossly unfair to England, which, because it has by far the largest number of registrants, carries a disproportionate financial burden in respect of supporting the rest of the UK – yet the registrants are not 'rewarded' by a corresponding increase in representation. The opposing argument is that this is about *equal* representation of the four countries concerned and that any form of proportional representation would disenfranchise the smaller countries.

In addition there is, of course, the issue of professional representation across the three professions of nursing, midwifery and health visiting. To an extent, the same arguments are deployed here. How do you ensure a system that ensures that the numerical minorities are not always 'coming from behind' and in danger of being out-voted. The debate has had two main facets over the years. This first is in relation to midwifery and how the unique nature of midwifery as a separate profession is ensured, within a statutory structure which regulates both professions. Secondly, there is the issue of wider representation within nursing. 'Nursing' is a single category within the Council elections. There are, however, those who have argued vehemently for specific representation from mental health, paediatrics and learning disabilities – not to mention occupational health, theatre nursing and so on and so on. Representation is always a fraught issue and probably always will be!

Principle of optimacy

Regulatory systems should provide and be restricted to those controls and restrictions necessary to achieve their objectives. This can be a real challenge. There can be a real temptation – particularly if those concerned are not truly signed up to, or do not really understand, the true meaning of working in the public interest – to be side-tracked into unnecessary intervention. There is certainly support for this view. I cannot count the number of times that practitioners with a problem have phoned the Council asking for explicit guidance in the form of written advice on an issue. They are often initially disconcerted when the response is to talk them through the principles and options, rather than to prescribe a specific solution. Fortunately most callers will soon appreciate that what is happening is a positive, facilitative process, designed to help them to apply principles to the specific subject with which they are grappling – e.g. an issue of confidentiality, poor colleague performance or accountability – in order for them to reach a way forward which is appropriate for their particular circumstances. In this way the practitioner has been supported, not instructed, and patient/client care hopefully enriched.

Principle of flexibility

Standards and processes of regulation should be sufficiently broad and flexible to achieve their objectives and at the same time permit freedom for innovation, growth and change. There is nothing more dispiriting for innovators than to be shackled by irrelevant and inappropriate rules and regulations. This poses a real problem for standard-setters in statutory bodies, bodies which by their very nature work comparatively slowly. It places an obligation upon them to ensure that the standards that are set in the first place are couched in such terms as to facilitate innovation and change, where that is appropriate. It will happen, however, that no matter how hard one tries, changes in the professional or educational context will outstrip the relevant legislation that underpins the standard. A good example of this is provided by the nurse training rules on the number of hours relating to the length of a programme leading to registration (which are based on the relevant European Union Directives). The nature of the rules is such that they did not accommodate the movement towards credit accumulation and transfer which was taking place in higher education. So, change the rules you say. That's fine, but even the simplest rule will take approximately 1 year to change, even assuming all goes well and there are no hitches at any stage in the process. And that's only in the United Kingdom. Changing legislation in the European Union is far more time-consuming and complex.

Contrast this with professional practice, where for nursing, there is no explicit, direct legislation and where the Council gives its guidance to practitioners through the form of advisory documents such as the *Code of Professional Conduct* or the *Scope of Professional Practice*. Yes, they still take time to prepare, but this can be a much quicker and more flexible process than using rules.

The skill is in knowing which aspects of the regulatory business *must* be enshrined in rules, e.g. professional conduct activity; which aspects are *best* enshrined in rules, such as some aspects of the education process; and which aspects are more effectively dealt through the use of other media, such as the *Code*.

Principle of efficiency and congruence

Regulatory systems should operate in the most efficient manner, ensuring coherence and coordination among their parts. This sounds easy and may be so, if one is building a new system from scratch. But that is not often the case. One rarely has the opportunity of writing on a truly blank page – usually someone has put in, if not the detail, at least a fair amount of text. This being the case it can be quite hard to ensure coherence and congruence.

In the UK, having a regulatory system which incorporates five bodies – the UKCC and four National Boards – presents unique challenges in ensuring congruence and coherence in the systems. And indeed these are not the only players. Let us look at it in a little more detail. The UKCC sets the broad parameters for professional standards – the body's skeleton, if you like. The National Boards then add flesh to the bones with their more detailed require-ments in relation to the nature of the professional programme and the standards to be achieved in relation to different aspects of the curriculum. It is, however, the staff in the actual higher education institution who design the curriculum and who deliver it on a daily basis. Another vitally important aspect is the clinical or practice setting, where individual students see the art and science of nursing and midwifery being put into effect.

So, with so many players involved it is very important to ensure con-gruence and coherence. This is a continuing challenge and an aspect of UK regulation which needs constant monitoring and is likely to need significant change.

Principle of universality

Regulatory systems should promote universal standards of performance and foster professional identity and mobility to the fullest extent compatible with local needs and circumstances. Universality of standards is of the most important, yet one of the most difficult, things to ensure. It can be difficult within an entity such as the UK, where the educational and the legal systems have significant differences within the four countries, let alone the organization and delivery of health care. Such differences can be even more difficult within a federated state, where standards may vary significantly from state to state. Think then how much greater this might be – and indeed is – from country to country. Let us take an immediate example, that of midwifery. In the UK it is accepted that midwifery is a separate profession from nursing, even though the majority of midwives (but by no means all) are also nurses. Midwives practise as autonomous practitioners, managing all aspects of normal deliveries themselves, either in the woman's home or in hospital. In some countries, notably parts of North America, midwifery of this nature is illegal – there are obstetric nurses, but their practice is under the supervision of obstetricians. Another nursing example: in many eastern European countries, nurses are trained to carry out doctor's orders – that is their role. There is no concept of autonomous nursing practice based on sound nursing research. Please don't misunderstand me – I am not necessarily criticising other systems, I am merely pointing out that they are significantly different and 'a nurse is a nurse is a nurse' is no more true than 'a doctor is a doctor is a doctor' or 'a lawyer is a lawyer is a lawyer'. Checks need to be made before one can assume the universality of practice and all possible steps should be taken to work towards coherent and consistent standards.

Principle of fairness

Regulatory systems should provide honest and just treatment for those parties concerned. Honest and just systems have to be designed to be transparent, with clear lines of accountability and clear and explicit routes of appeal for the public and professionals alike

This applies to all aspects of the regulatory activity, whether it be the setting of standards for professional education, entry to the register (from within the UK, the European Union or elsewhere), maintaining registration or professional conduct. All those involved in the process have to be clear as to what is expected of them in all respects and lack of success – whether it be for an overseas nurse or midwife seeking registration with the UKCC, or a nurse or midwife who has been removed from the register by the professional conduct committee – has to be made explicit with clear and demonstrable reasons for the decision. There should also be clear and visible appeal processes, so that individuals who feel that they have not been well served can seek some form of review.

The public have a right to know what the regulatory body is doing, on their behalf, in the public interest. This information has to be available in clear and unambiguous language with identified routes for contact, advice and/or complaint.

The somewhat secretive nature of traditional professional decision-making in the past – where it was difficult to get access to good, clear information and explanations were never, or rarely, given for the decisions reached – no longer serves the more articulate public and the individual professionals of the 1990s and beyond.

Principle of interprofessional equality and compatibility

In standards and processes regulatory systems should recognize the equality and interdependence of professions. No professionals – certainly not in the health service – practise in a vacuum. Good quality patient and client care is dependent on cooperative and facilitative working between the professionals involved. This is likely to involve an ever greater range of individuals, representing, for example, hospital medicine, physiotherapy, occupational therapy, management, community nursing staff and general practice, to name but a few. Cooperation with other professions, such as social work, also becomes ever more relevant as the lines between health and social care become ever more blurred. The emphasis on teamwork makes some fairly radical changes to old patterns of status and relative role and can take some major adjustments on the part of all the staff concerned.

Providing that all the parties concerned have appropriate and adequate opportunities to get together to talk things through and decide between them what is best for their patient and clients, then improved care should result, with increased consumer and professional satisfaction. Such discussions, however, will only be successful if they are premised on interprofessional equality and respect and not based on traditional hierarchies.

This section has looked at broad issues associated with professional regulation. It is now necessary to turn to the individual professional and explore their role within the regulatory framework.

ACCOUNTABILITY – ANSWERING FOR YOUR ACTIONS

Accountability is a complex and multifaceted subject. Different commentators will approach it in differing ways and offer different models or frameworks within which to consider the relevant issues. This serves to enrich the debate and allows us all to select a view, or views, that most comfortably sits with our own. What is in no doubt is that individual professionals have an accountability to their individual professional peers, their team/department, the employing organization, their statutory body and/or professional organization and society. They also have a wider accountability which embraces individual and organizational users of their service, potential users, the community, interest groups, tax payers and society and the government.

Where can we get help on the issue of accountability? The *Oxford Dictionary and Thesaurus* (1995) helps only a little. Accountability is defined as being 'responsible, required to account for one's conduct, answerable, liable or chargeable'.

Eraut (1996, unpublished lecture) described three conceptual dimensions of accountability, as follows:

- *a moral dimension* – that is, accountability to anyone who is affected by one's action

- *a contractual dimension* – that owed to one's employer
- *a professional dimension* – to oneself, colleagues and the organization.

His analysis of the issues associated with accountability concludes that contractual accountability should be weak and flexible. Moral and professional accountability will then be strong. On the other hand, where contractual responsibility is too strong then the punitive nature of the contract will uncouple the individuals concerned from their professional and moral obligations – to the detriment of innovative, compassionate and considered practice. I think this is an insightful and helpful analysis.

Other frameworks suggest four key elements of accountability: that of accountability to the public (criminal law), accountability to the patient (civil law), accountability to the employer (contractual law) and accountability to the profession (professional 'law').

Lavin (1995, unpublished) suggested that for a professional to be considered legally accountable, they need four specific things:

- a degree of autonomy
- a freedom to act or practise in accordance with training and education
- the use of judgement and the power to act on it
- a skill in the art and profession.

These are important issues and each professional on the register will need to consider in what respects they meet these criteria in the exercise of their professional practice. It is likely that the answers will vary considerably from person to person and from place to place. This will depend on, amongst other things, the age, personality, experience, competence and confidence of the individual practitioner, whether they have done any additional education, the 'culture' (trusting or blaming) in which they work, local policies and the management structure in which they operate. Whatever the answers, it is important that individual registrants think the matter through for themselves and clarify in their own minds what their position is. There is plenty of help available, not least from the UKCC.

The UKCC's original document on accountability (UKCC 1989) states that 'accountability is an integral part of professional practice, since, in the course of that practice, the individual has to make judgements in a wide variety of circumstances and be answerable for those judgements'.

It goes on to say that the principles against which accountability should be exercised are as follows (UKCC 1989):

- The interest of the patient or client are paramount.
- Professional accountability must be exercised in such a manner as to ensure the primacy of the interests of the patient or clients is respected and must not be overridden by those of the professions or their practitioners.
- The exercise of accountability requires the practitioner to seek to achieve and maintain high standards.

- Advocacy on behalf of patients and clients is an essential feature of the exercise of accountability by a professional practitioner.
- The role of the other persons in the delivery of health care to patients and clients must be recognized and respected, provided the first principle above is honoured.
- Public trust and confidence in the professions are dependent upon its practitioners being seen to exercise their accountability responsibly.
- Each registered nurse, midwife or health visitor must be able to justify any action or decision not to act taken in the course of his/her professional practice.

In the *Guidelines for Professional Practice* (UKCC 1996), which replaced, amongst others, the original document on accountability, there is a very real and welcome effort to make the concept of accountability even more understandable to those who often struggle with the realities of it on a daily basis. Practitioners are reminded that they 'hold a position of responsibility and other people rely on you. You are professionally accountable to the UKCC, as well as having a contractual responsibility to your employers and accountability to the law for your actions.'

Code of Professional Conduct

The document goes on to remind practitioners that it is their code of conduct (UKCC 1992a) which sets out their accountability in detail. The *Code of Professional Conduct* is probably the most important document ever put out by the UKCC. Judging from the distances it travels, the places where it is quoted and the number of times it is expressly acknowledged in the production of similar codes in both other countries and other professions (either explicitly or by imitation, as in 'imitation being the sincerest form of flattery'), that is also what a lot of other people and professions think. It is no exaggeration to say that it is a truly universal document and its wise counsel informs professionals all over the world.

Reg Pyne, the prime mover of the *Code*, described it as (Pyne 1994, unpublished work):

a clarion call to professional practitioners to be professional, thinking not only of the short term, but also strategically about those who will require professional care in the future and of how that will be provided. It is a plea to each and every practitioner to be an agent of positive change focused on high standards and good outcomes, rather than a victim of change decreed by others. Those who place themselves in your care deserve no less.

I make no apologies for repeating parts of this important document. It starts with the following clear and unequivocal statement:

Each registered nurse, midwife and health visitor shall act, at all times, in such a manner as to safeguard and promote the interests of individual patients and clients; serve the interests of society; justify public trust and confidence and uphold and enhance the good standing and reputations of the professions.

This leaves no-one in any doubt, at least in principle, about the range and nature of their responsibilities. It goes on to give more guidance and this is where the first and last mention of accountability by name is found – in the statement at the beginning of the *Code*, which is the basis for *every* subsequent clause, the stem of the *Code*, which states (my emphasis):

As a registered nurse, midwife or health visitor, you are *personally accountable* for your practice and, in the exercise of *your* professional accountability must: ...

In other words, every element of the code is based on the concept of the individual's personal accountability. To labour the point beyond reasonable doubt – no-one else can ever take responsibility for *your* actions as a registered nurse, midwife or health visitor. It is never sufficient justification to say that you were told to do something by another, if, in the light of your knowledge and experience (and that is both your actual knowledge and the knowledge you would be 'reasonably' expected to have, for the position you hold, in the light of your qualifications, experience and responsibility), the action was inappropriate, dangerous, or not in the best interests of your patients and clients. So, there is no such thing as accountability by proxy. Neither can accountability be considered an optional extra, to be activated or discarded as you see fit.

The *Code* goes on to set out all the ways in which you demonstrate your accountability as a professional. It makes it clear that you must always act in such a way as to promote and safeguard the interests and well-being of your patients and clients. You must make sure that you do nothing which will cause them harm. You must keep up to date, and also not do things for which you have not been properly prepared. You are required to work collaboratively with other people and professionals in the patient's best interests. You must maintain the dignity of those for whom you care and never abuse the position of trust into which your status as a registered nurse, midwife or health visitor has placed you. And so it goes on, clause after clause, key statement after key statement, setting out the profession's expectations of you as a registered professional. Indeed, this is the template against which your performance or behaviour will be judged, should you ever be called to account for your actions.

This concept of professional accountability in nursing and midwifery is not universal and, indeed, is one of the most challenging elements in the movement of professionals from one country to another. There are still many countries in the world where other professions, virtually always doctors, take total responsibility for the actions of nurses and midwives (if there are any). In these situations, the doctors will give orders to the nurses and expect them to be obeyed without question. The activity of nursing, in these situations, hardly meets the various criteria necessary for being a profession, which includes, among other things, at least a degree of personal and professional autonomy.

The UKCC, having nailed its colours firmly to the mast in the *Code of Professional Conduct*, in terms of how it wished to regulate the professions –

as individual, accountable professionals – then took another major step forward, at the same time as the PREP project was underway. This was the production of the *Scope of Professional Practice* document (UKCC 1992b).

Scope of Professional Practice

The *Scope of Professional Practice* grows from the *Code of Conduct* and it was no coincidence that the third edition of the *Code* and the new *Scope* document were published at the same time. Indeed, they were not only published, but also mailed to every one of the individual registered nurses, midwives and health visitors on the UKCC's professional register. It is a document of immense significance, yet – as is often the case with matters of such importance – it is actually only a statement, or collection of statements, of the obvious. The obvious to one person, however, is not obvious to all and frequently does need to be stated and unpicked.

What was the background to the production of the document? As is frequently the case, this was complex and multifaceted. One of the most important issues was the notion of 'extended role' which was in place at the time. This was promoted by the government health departments and whilst originally promulgated in 1977, had been reiterated as comparatively recently as 1989. In essence, this was the idea of only being allowed to add to the skills learnt during pre-registration education, by undertaking a 'course' and having an appropriate 'certificate' signed to signify an individual's competence, in relation to a specific task. Whilst the intention behind the idea was no doubt sound, and presumably was based on the principle of wishing to ensure patient safety, what it did was to create a practical situation which frequently became, in effect, a nonsense. Experienced staff who moved from one place of employment to another often had to wait months to do the appropriate course at their new workplace – only to find that they were repeating what they had already been doing for years. This approach resulted in a significant waste and duplication of both human and financial resources. Far more important, however, was the stultifying approach on professional practice of having to acquire a certificate for each new task learned, rather than working to a set of principles which could underpin all aspects of an individual's informed and accountable professional practice. Such an approach in fact *limited*, rather than extended, practice. It was also, in a sense, a hypocritical approach to professional practice, in that it was often expected that the very tasks in question would be undertaken in an emergency situation, yet not in others.

There were also a range of other factors influencing the call for change and the need for a more mature, accountable form of professional practice, in order to better meet the needs of patients and clients. Not least amongst these factors was the ever increasing amount of knowledge and range of new skills needed in order to practise safely and effectively, in the light of rapidly changing technology and the new bodies of knowledge arising from research activity. There were also significant changes to professional practice, with a much more interactive and participative approach being used between those being cared for and those doing the caring. The changing patterns of service delivery also had, and continues to have, a significant effect on practice.

Changing skill mix and the changing boundaries of practice between professions, particularly between nursing and midwifery, and medicine were also important issues. It was frequently alleged that the initiatives in relation to junior doctors' hours influenced the UKCC's decisions in relation to freeing up the practice of its registrants, but this was emphatically not the case.

One of the most important factors requiring a change in professional practice is the increasing knowledge and expectations of those for whom we care. The volume and range of information now available to many, be it through the medium of newspapers, radio, television or the Internet, is vast and increasing daily. Our patients and clients are better informed and more articulate than they have ever been and rightly expect, and if necessary demand, a good level of service. Consumer charters of all kinds have raised expectations – even if not always appropriately – and placed new pressures on professionals to deliver care differently.

There are also the unrelenting pressures of diminishing budgets within an increasingly cash-strapped service. Managers have to look for ways of delivering quality care at a reduced, or at least a contained, cost. It is important that professionals play their part in such activity – not to reduce the service but to honestly and openly examine their own practice to see if there are things that could be changed without a reduction in quality or standards of care.

So, to recap, there were a myriad of reasons in the early 1990s why it was necessary to move away from the existing situation to one which was designed specifically to free up professional practice and give practitioners the tools to take their practice forward, safely, effectively and, where appropriate, imaginatively, into the next century.

Having looked a little at the background to the production of the *Scope of Professional Practice* let us turn to the document itself.

Principles for adjusting the scope of professional practice

It is not my intention to look at the whole *Scope* document in detail. You may well have already done that in the course of your work, or indeed you may be inspired to do so as a result of reading this chapter. But I would like to look at the principles for adjusting the scope of practice because they are just so important. My personal view is that a sound understanding of the principles is all that you really need. The rest of the document is very helpful, but the essence lies in the principles – grasp these and your practice can be transformed!

The principles are, of course, based on the UKCC *Code of Conduct*, as this is where the *Scope* has its origins. In particular, it is based upon the emphasis which the *Code* places on the acquisition of knowledge and skill, together with the exercise of responsibility and personal professional accountability. In essence, the principles give the template against which any individual practitioner, or group of practitioners, can consider any changes to their existing professional practice. Providing you can satisfy yourself, and if necessary others, that you have satisfied the principles set out below, then you can be assured that you are adjusting your scope of practice appropriately.

The registered nurse, midwife or health visitor:

• *Must be satisfied that each aspect of practice is directed to meeting the needs and serving the interests of patients or clients.* This is the essence of expanding your scope of practice. If, in expanding and enhancing the role of the registered practitioner, you are not more effectively serving those for whom you care, then the expansion in your practice has not been for the right reasons and should be reconsidered. It is, of course, possible to adjust your scope of practice for all sorts of reasons. It could be through a misguided sense of professional aggrandizement – to enhance professional practice in the eyes of others. It could be out of a genuine wish to help other professions – doing the i.v. drugs, for example, to save getting the junior medical staff out of bed in the middle of the night. It could be, unintentionally or otherwise, for your own self-aggrandizement – to be seen to be doing the 'glamorous' or high-tech activities that traditionally have been preciously associated with other professions, usually medicine. It could be that you have been told to do it, in order to save money and/or staff. Whatever the reason, if the patient/client is not firmly in the centre of the activity, resulting in an improvement in their care, then it is not an appropriate reason for an expansion of practice. If you can answer this question honestly, then you should have no doubt that what you are doing is right, providing you can also satisfy yourself that you also meet the other principles.

• *Must endeavour always to achieve, maintain and develop knowledge and skill and take steps to remedy any relevant deficits in order to effectively and appropriately to meet the needs of patients and clients.* I said that the document set out statements of the obvious and indeed it does! There is an imperative upon us all to be sure, as far as is reasonably possible, that we not only have the necessary knowledge at any given time to care for our patients/clients, but that we constantly nurture and replenish that knowledge on a regular basis. It is very easy to get into practice ruts and routines and to do something because it 'has always been done this way' – custom and practice is a powerful mantra with which to stifle innovation and change. Can you be sure that you are in possession of the best, most up-to-date knowledge relating to a particular nursing or medical problem? Are you aware of the most recent relevant research in the particular field, are you confident that you know the effects of this particular disease on this particular patient? Are there new techniques that could be used to make things better for your patient or client? It is your responsibility to know these things. Fortunately you are rarely alone. There are usually others who can help you gather the information, but make sure that you deal with it systematically – don't all read the same professional journal; make sure that between you, you cover all sources likely to be of help.

• *Must honestly acknowledge any limits of personal knowledge and skill and take steps to remedy any relevant deficits in order effectively and appropriately to meet the needs of patients and clients.* Of course, the flip side of needing to know as much as possible about the care you are giving is to realize that none of us are omnipotent and we cannot possibly know everything. You are expected to have a reasonable knowledge of your field of care, and if you profess to be an expert, either implicitly or explicitly, by virtue of your title or your role, you will be expected to have knowledge in excess of that possessed by the 'average' practitioner. However, sooner or later you will come up against something you don't know about and you must say so. It is a denial of professional accountability to pretend to know – or do – something for which you have not been properly prepared and for which you do not have the necessary knowledge or skills base.

• *Must ensure that any enlargement or adjustment of the scope of personal professional practice must be achieved without compromising or fragmenting existing aspects of professional practice and care and that the requirements of the* Code of Professional Conduct *are satisfied throughout the whole area of practice.* This is an important principle. It is very easy, when very busy and taking on additional activity, to end up fragmenting care, rather than enhancing it. It requires considerable clarity of thinking about the proper and appropriate roles of all the individuals concerned – nurses and midwives, other health care professionals, patients/clients, support staff and carers. If you are to take on something new, is that to be at the expense of something else, and if so, what? Are you sure that you are relinquishing the right thing(s)? Is there someone else who can take on what you no longer have time for? If so, who, and are they, or can they be, properly prepared?

• *Must recognize and honour the personal accountability borne for all aspects of professional practice.* An adjusted scope of professional practice requires a clear understanding of professional accountability. If you, as a registered nurse or midwife, are adjusting your scope of practice – regardless of who has been undertaking that aspect of care before – then you remain accountable for all your actions in your enhanced role. It is never acceptable, should anything be questioned, to say that you only did something because you were told to do so, or that another is 'taking responsibility' for your actions. You and you alone will be called to account for what you do.

• *Must, in serving the interests of patients and clients and the wider interests of society avoid any inappropriate delegation to others which compromises those interests.* I think that the art of delegation is one of the most complex and demanding skills needed by registered practitioners at the turn of the 20th century. The huge changes which have come about as a result of cost-cutting activity, skill-mix initiatives and re-profiling alone, and the resultant dilution of registered staff, have placed heavy responsibilities on those who coordinate professional care. And after all, who is it, amongst all the health care professionals, who is present with the patient 24 hours a day – it is the nurses. This is not the voice of professional tribalism speaking, but a matter of observable and measurable fact. Other health care professionals have important roles but they are intermittent in their nature – it is the nurse who remains when the others have gone. Given that it is not possible, or indeed appropriate, for nurses (and this is more of a nursing issue than a midwifery one at the moment, although that may well change) to deliver every aspect of what can be considered to be nursing care personally, then effective delegation is vital. Delegation can be activated in all directions and requires a clear understanding of, amongst other things, the particular patient/client, their problems, their carers, the stage at which they are being cared for, and the others that are available within the team and their particular skills and competencies. Delegation is an issue which I believe can push professional accountability to its limits and often may well result in unpalatable decisions, depending on individual circumstances.

CONCLUSION

This chapter may well have tried to do too much, as the issues under consideration are so complex and challenging. I hope, however, that there has been a logical progression of ideas and issues within the context of the changing face of professional regulation. The individuals on the UKCC register have been regulated on the basis of an increased understanding of the true meaning and implications of professional accountability and trust. To see how such an approach influenced the way in which the UKCC has managed one of its biggest challenges of the 1990s – that of setting a framework for professional education and practice after registration – please read on.

REFERENCES

Affara F A, Styles M M 1992 Nursing regulation guidebook: from principle to power. International Council of Nurses, Geneva
Davies C 1995 Gender and the professional predicament in nursing. Open University Press, Buckingham
Department of Health 1993 Changing childbirth – report of the Expert Maternity Group. HMSO, London
HMSO 1989 The Nurses, Midwives and Health Visitors rules (Registered Fever Nurses and Nurse Training Rules) Approval Order 1989. Statutory Instrument No 1456. HMSO, London

International Council of Nurses 1985 Report on the regulation of nursing. A report for the present, a position for the future. ICN, Geneva *Based on a project report by Margretta M Styles*

Pyne R 1997 Professional discipline in nursing, midwifery and health visiting. Blackwell Science, Oxford

UKCC 1989 Exercising accountability. UKCC, London (out of print)

UKCC 1992 Code of professional conduct. UKCC, London

UKCC 1992 Scope of professional practice UKCC, London

UKCC 1993 Midwives rules. UKCC, London

UKCC 1996 Guidelines for professional practice. UKCC, London

The origins, role and functions of the UKCC

Who controls the past, controls the future. Who controls the present, controls the past.

(*Nineteen Eighty-Four*, George Orwell)

INTRODUCTION

To make sense of the PREP story, a working understanding of the role and functions of the UKCC is necessary. Regrettably, and no doubt for a whole variety of reasons, there are very few registered nurses, midwives and health visitors who really understand how the UKCC works on their behalf, in the public interest. This, sadly, was incontrovertibly demonstrated by the most recent elections to the Council in the summer of 1997, when only 13% of the potential 640 000 plus electorate bothered to voted for the new Council – i.e. those individuals who will be responsible for setting the standards for their professions for the next 5 years. I hope that this chapter will help to redress that balance in some small way and give you an idea of how the Council came into being and how it works and what its relationships are with other bodies. I would suggest that, even if you are not keen on professional history, you might like to, at the least, read the section on how the UKCC works, even if you don't want to wade through the rest. Personally, I think the history is fascinating, but then you already know that I am biased!

What this chapter sets out to do, therefore, is to give a brief history of the Council and its work prior to the PREP initiative. It also sets the work of the Council into context, particularly in relation to other statutory and professional bodies, such as the National Boards for Nursing , Midwifery and Health Visiting and the professional organizations and trade unions. It also looks at how the Council works with government departments, the other statutory bodies in the health sector, the purchasers and providers of health and education, employers and, very importantly, consumers.

THE ORIGINS OF THE UKCC

In 1972, the Committee on Nursing, chaired by Professor Asa Briggs (Committee of Nursing 1972), reported. It recommended a new statutory structure to bring the nursing and midwifery professions closer together and to link this development with the forthcoming integration of the National Health Service. The committee had ideas for a structure which was to bring together the different countries of the United Kingdom and the different groups involved. These ideas were modified over time, during the long process of discussions with those who would be affected. The UKCC and four National Boards for Nursing, Midwifery and Health Visiting were finally established as a result of The Nurses, Midwives and Health Visitors Act 1979 (HMSO 1979). The Act was passed in the closing days of the then Labour government and only just made it on to the statute books before the government fell. The bodies existed in 'shadow' form from 1981 until the 'appointed day' of 1 July 1983, which is when the 1979 Act came into effect. The 1979 Act was subsequently amended in 1992 by an Act of the same name (HMSO 1992). The 1979 and 1992 Acts were then amalgamated in 1997, with no major change of content, into The Nurses, Midwives and Health Visitors Act 1997 (The Stationary Office 1997). As was pointed out in references in the preface, convention requires that it is always the latest legislation that is referenced. So, unless otherwise stated, from now on, when referring to the Act of Parliament which deal with nursing, midwifery and health visiting, it will be the 1997 Act, unless one of the earlier Acts is specifically mentioned by date. This may cause some confusion, as it was necessary to change the numbering of the sections of the 1979 and 1992 Acts when they were consolidated in 1997.

When looking at the legislation with the benefit of hindsight, it is easy to identify a number of flaws within it. However, at the time, and given the vested interests involved, it was in reality a masterpiece of drafting, compromise and tact. For the first time, nursing, midwifery and health visiting, in the four countries of the UK, were united in one statutory structure with a remit for managing both pre- and post-registration education and practice.

The new statutory structure replaced the previous nine statutory and training bodies, which had between them dealt separately with nursing, midwifery, health visiting, district nursing, pre-registration education and post-basic education in England and Wales, Scotland and Northern Ireland. The outgoing bodies were:

- The General Nursing Council for England and Wales
- The General Nursing Council for Scotland
- The Northern Ireland Council for Nurses and Midwives
- The Central Midwives Board for England and Wales
- The Central Midwives Board for Scotland

- The Panel of Assessors for District Nurse Training
- The Council for the Education and Training of Health Visitors
- The Joint Board of Clinical Nursing Studies (England and Wales)
- Committee for Clinical Nursing Studies (Scotland).

The shadow days

The task of drawing together the roles and functions of these bodies was, as one might imagine, complex and time-consuming, as they all had different systems. For example, the GNC (E and W) had computerized its registration records, while other bodies had not. Some of the bodies registered people for life on payment of an initial registration fee, while some others charged no initial registration fee but did charge annual registration fees. Others still did not charge fees, since they were deficit-funded by the government, an arrangement which died with the coming into operation of the 1979 Act in July 1983 (HMSO 1979). The UKCC was therefore starting its life with a slender and confused financial base and was operating on the proverbial shoestring. Confusion was also apparent in relation to the records of the various bodies. Some people were on the records of more than one of the bodies, though they may have changed their name and achieved new qualifications which were recorded in only one country of the UK. There were also significant differences in the ways the bodies worked. Some of the organizations met in public, including hearings with a view to removal from the register, while others did not.

The fact that there was not, at that time, any central, comprehensive and up-to-date register made it extremely difficult for the UKCC to meet the requirements of the new Act, which was to conduct an election in order to elect the majority of the members of the new National Boards. During the shadow period, from 1981 to 1983, the very few staff then employed by the Council were busily employed tramping up and down the UK addressing meetings, in order to persuade nurses, midwives and health visitors to opt into the electoral register. Each opting-in form then had to be checked against the registers of the extant, but soon to disappear, registration bodies to justify their inclusion in the electoral role. This helped to match the records of many people who were registered, for the same or different qualifications, in more than one country, or with more than one body. One unexpected – and beneficial in terms of public protection – by-product was that this process brought to the surface for prosecution a number of people in professional practice who did not have the qualifications they purported to have, or, indeed were not who or what they purported to be!

The UKCC staff and members had to work hard to ensure that this comparatively brief shadow period was used wisely and well, in order to prepare the ground and build the foundations on which it would be standing for years to come. A number of working groups were established to explore both the existing bodies' core activities and the new legal responsibilities and powers of the new Council; these are detailed below.

Working Group 1 was charged with preparing an electoral scheme to allow elections to take place to each of the National Boards (there were no direct elections to the Council at this time). This is how the majority of the board members were put into place. The remaining members were to be appointed by the Secretary of State. A full evaluation of the scheme was undertaken at the time, in order to inform future elections.

Working Group 2 was established to decide which qualifications were to be recorded on the new single professional register, and what the means should be of maintaining and updating the register and associated policy questions that arose from those decisions. Some of the questions that were posed for resolution included the following:

• *Should there be an upper age limit?* The final decision was that there should be no age limit. This is still the case, although since 1995, of course, individuals have to meet the PREP requirements in order to remain registered, regardless of age.

• *Should information on academic and professional qualifications be added to the register?* The final decision was that it should be those qualifications relevant to professional practice which should be registered, so professional qualifications were registered, academic qualifications were not

• *What conditions, if any, should there be made on entitlement to practise?* The final decision was that there should be no conditions on practice made at that time, as it was such a complex issue, but it would be an issue to return to once the time was right. Periodic registration was, of course, subsequently introduced, followed by the PREPP initiative.

• *Should there be periodic fees?* The final decision was that this should be introduced as soon as it could be done.

It was at this stage that the decision was taken to have two levels of nurse, to reflect those who had been on either the register or the roll of the previous bodies and who had, unsurprisingly, been known as registered and enrolled nurses (see the section on parts of the register in the preface). Individuals were to be known, therefore, as first and second level nurses. With hindsight, this decision in relation to terminology was, I believe, most unfortunate and unintentionally divisive. 'Second level' was certainly felt by many enrolled nurses to be a judgmental term and imply 'second class'. In practice, the terms 'registered' and 'enrolled' are still frequently used, as it is a familiar and well understood shorthand. It does not, however, accurately reflect the position of 'enrolled' nurses, as they are, of course, *registered* with the UKCC and are therefore entitled to call themselves registered nurses, providing they make it clear, like everyone on the register is required to do, what type of qualification they hold.

Working Group 3 had the difficult task of looking at issues to do with education and training. The main issues discussed were the shape and framework of pre-registration courses, which would lead individuals on to the professional register, the proportion of support staff needed to help the registered practitioners, the role of the student nurse, midwife or health visitor, employment legislation and the requirements for colleges of nursing and midwifery. Active debate on the issues, rather than reactive comments on prescriptive recommendations, was encouraged at this stage, in order to give as many people as possible a chance to comment on the very significant issues that were being raised. The final recommendations included the following:

- There should be one single standard qualification as a registered nurse, without prejudice to enrolled nurses who were to be encouraged to convert and who could continue in practice.
- Registration (i.e. not qualification alone) would mark the entry of the nurse or midwife into the profession.
- Students would be in controlled learning environments and were not to be in a position of having professional accountability for care.
- Colleges of Nursing and Midwifery were to be established.
- There should be total funding of students.

At this stage, the Council decided to establish a 2 year project to look at education and training requirements. This subsequently became known as Project 2000 and is dealt with in more detail in the next chapter.

Working Group 4 was established to look at the important and complex issues associated with what was then known as professional discipline and is now known as professional conduct. The group was remitted to formulate a clear view of the purpose of professional discipline and to devise mechanisms for this function to be carried out effectively within the new statutory structure. The key recommendations from the group were that there should be:

- legal handling of allegations and convictions
- representation at hearings
- committees to deal with the disciplinary process
- fitness to practice linked to health or incapacity
- voluntary removal or suspension from the register
- appeals.

The professional conduct rules were subsequently drafted and came into force on 1 July 1983 (HMSO 1983).

Working Group 5 looked at the establishment of the standing and joint committees (i.e. joint between the Council and National Boards) and also the discretionary – or additional – committees needed to help the Council fulfil its functions within the legislation. Initially the Midwifery Committee, Health Visiting Joint Committee and Finance Committee were established. In addition, an Education Policy Advisory Committee and a District Nursing Joint Committee were also set up.

Working Group 6 was tasked with managing the handover of functions from the old, outgoing statutory and training bodies to the new bodies in the new statutory structure. The members were required to decide what organizational/management structure, manpower requirements, transfer of staff and accommodation were needed. They considered, among other things:

- the date for the handover of functions
- organization and staffing plans for the whole organization
- financial systems
- personnel policies
- computer functions
- communications with the extant bodies and their staff.

After consultation, a range of policies were agreed and the handover date was confirmed as 30 June 1983.

Working Group 7 was required to 'advise on the transfer of properties held by the existing bodies'. Two main areas of work were identified, one relating to the estimation of future accommodation needs and the other to the existing resources of the extant bodies. It was agreed that the new UK Central Council would take over the property of the General Nursing Council for England and Wales in Portland Place, London.

Thus were the foundations gradually built. The recommendations from the various groups were agreed by the shadow council, with or without modification, after consultation. As a result, the necessary legislation could be prepared in order to be ready for the 'appointed day', i.e. the day that the new structure came into effect.

The nursing, midwifery and health visiting professions, I believe, have every reason to be grateful for the foresight and vision of those who spent so many of their own hours planning for all our futures.

Shadow into substance

As we have seen, the new statutory structure set up by the 1979 Act consisted of a UK Central Council and four National Boards for England, Scotland, Northern Ireland and Wales. The Council and National Boards are therefore statutory bodies (i.e. set up as a result of legislation). As their functions are, in different ways, to regulate the profession, they are also regulatory bodies. They are, therefore, properly described as statutory, regulatory bodies. Their functions are interdependent and they work together in a collegiate, not a hierarchical, manner.

THE FUNCTIONS OF THE UKCC

The functions of the UKCC were originally set out in Section 2 of The Nurses, Midwives and Health Visitors Act 1979, as follows:

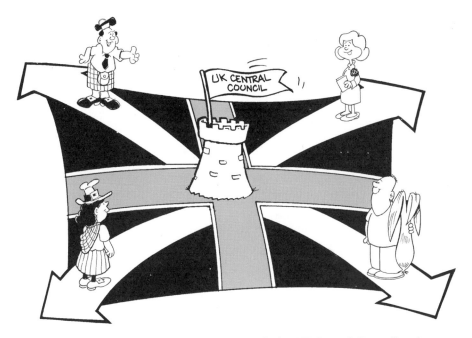

'... the new statutory structure consisted of a UK Central Council and four National Boards.'

2(1) The principal functions of the Central Council shall be to establish and improve standards of training and professional conduct for nurses, midwives and health visitors.

(2) The Council shall ensure that the standards of training they establish are such as to meet any Community obligation of the United Kingdom.

(3) The Council shall by rules determine the conditions of a person's being admitted to training, and the kind and standard of training to be undertaken, with a view to registration.

(4) The rules may also make provision with respect to the kind and standard of further training available to persons who are already registered.

(5) The powers of the Council shall include that of providing, in such a manner as it thinks fit, advice for nurses, midwives and health visitors on standards of professional conduct.

(6) In the discharge of its functions the Council shall have proper regard for the interests of all groups within the professions, including those with minority representation.

The 1992 Act retained, unchanged, the functions of the Council, with the addition of the word 'content' in clause 2(3), so that it now read 'the kind, *content* and standard of training'. The 1997 Act contained no changes in relation to the functions of the Council.

THE FUNCTIONS OF THE NATIONAL BOARDS

Section 6 of The Nurses, Midwives and Health Visitors Act 1979 set out the functions of the four National Boards as follows:

6(1)   The National Boards shall in England, Wales, Scotland and Northern Ireland respectively –

    (a)   provide, or arrange for others to provide, at institutions approved by the Board –

        (i)   courses of training with a view to enabling persons to qualify for registration as nurses, midwives or health visitors or for the recording of additional qualifications in the register, and

        (ii)   courses of further training for those already registered;

    (b)   ensure that such courses meet the requirements of the Central Council as to their kind, content and standard;

    (c)   hold, or arrange for others to hold, such examinations as are necessary to enable persons to satisfy requirements for registration or to obtain additional qualifications;

    (d)   collaborate with the Council in the promotion of improved training methods; and

    (e)   carry out investigations of alleged misconduct, with a view to proceedings before the central Council or a committee of the Council for a person to be removed from the register.

The 1992 Act removed the investigative function from the National Boards and placed it with the UKCC. Paragraph (e) was therefore replaced with the following:

    (e)   perform such other functions relating to nurses, midwives or health visitors as the Secretary of State may by order prescribe.

The 1992 Act (HMSO 1992) also changed the election system. Elections for the first two 5 year terms of the Council's office were to the four National Boards, and the National Boards then nominated some of their members to the Council (those members then being in membership of a National Board and the Council concurrently). After 1992, elections took place – and still do – directly onto the Council. National Boards members are appointed by the Secretary of State for Health.

The 1997 Act was, in essence, a consolidation measure and contained no major changes with regard to function of the Council and the National Boards.

REVIEW OF THE FUNCTIONS OF THE COUNCIL AND NATIONAL BOARDS

In March 1997, a fundamental review of the functions of the Council and National Boards was announced. Announcing it, Stephen Dorrell, then Secretary of State for Health, said:

There are 650 000 registered nurses, midwives and health visitors in the United Kingdom, representing the backbone of our National Health Services. It is essential that their framework for professional self-regulation should be responsive to continuing changes in public expectations and in the delivery of services.'

He went on to say that it is government policy to regularly review non-departmental public bodies. Although the UKCC does not fall into that category, the National Boards do, and as the legislation describes an integrated structure involving all five bodies, clearly any review must include them all.

The terms of reference for the review were, Mr Dorrell said:

'... to review the roles, functions and organization of the five statutory bodies established under the Nurses, Midwives and Health Visitors Act 1979 (as amended 1992) to ensure that they are adequately accountable to Parliament for the exercise of their statutory functions, and their use of public funds generally and that they continue to operate efficiently, effectively and economically. The review will examine the structure and constitution, interrelationship; functions and policy objectives of each body; and their relationships with government, employers, educational institutions, professional organizations and the public. It will make recommendations to the four UK health departments.'

The review will have regard to (press release, Department of Health 1997):

- the distinction between the responsibilities, roles and funding of the UKCC and National Boards
- the responsibility of the statutory bodies to the public and the nursing professions
- the need to distinguish, in relation to any proposals for change, between those which can be implemented within existing arrangements, and those requiring legislative change, and to identify any resource implications.

At the time of writing this book, the review team had commenced its work and was due to make recommendations at about the same time as this book will be published, in the summer of 1998. Whatever the recommendations, after consultation, it is likely that significant changes will be made to the existing statutory structure, and those structures described here will eventually take their place within the overall fabric of the history of the nursing, midwifery and health visiting professions. This makes a knowledge and understanding of the existing framework – warts and all – even more important for those of us who are currently part of it, those who were part of it, and also for those who may be part of a different future.

THE WAY THE UKCC WORKS

So having looked at the establishment of the Council and its formal legislative functions, it is worth taking a quick look at how the work actually gets done in practice. How does the UKCC actually carry out its functions?

The Council itself consists of a number of members who, since 1992, have been directly elected to the Council on a 5-yearly basis. As I explained earlier in this chapter, prior to 1992, the elections were to the National Boards, who then subsequently each nominated seven of their members to sit on the Council – four nurses, two midwives and one health visitor from each country. From 1983 to 1993 the Council had a total of 45 members – 28 from the National Boards and the remaining 17 as Secretary of State appointments. From 1993, to accommodate the increased workload associated with taking on the investigative functions previously held by the Boards, Council membership increased to 60. Forty members are now directly elected, by the professions, to the Council – seven nurses, two midwives and one health visitor each, from England, Scotland, Northern Ireland and Wales. The additional 20 members are Secretary of State appointments, chosen to supplement the knowledge and experience of the elected members. Once appointed, the Council acts as a body corporate (and is referred to as a corporate body in the singular – in other words, the Council is an 'it', not a 'them' when referring to the Council as a whole).

Council meetings are held every 2 months, but a huge amount of work is done outside the Council meetings themselves, both in order to inform the debate at the meetings and also to progress work that does not need the attention of the whole Council. Significant debate and decision-making takes place in the committees and most members of Council will be on one or more committee. The committees have changed over time to accommodate the varying needs of the organization, but at the time of writing are the Midwifery Committee and the Finance Committee (both statutory committees), the Joint Education Committee (i.e. joint between nursing, including community nursing, and midwifery) and the Nursing and Community

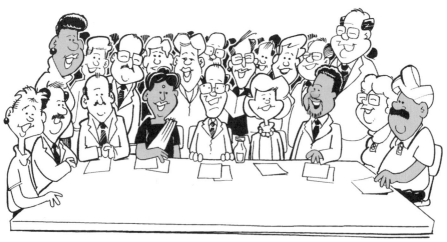

'Council meetings are held every two months.'

Health Care Nursing Committee. All Council members are potentially members of the Professional Conduct or Health committees, as part of either the preliminary proceedings activity or the professional conduct or health hearings themselves.

A wide range of work is also done through the medium of task groups, which are designed to be small, focused, time-limited and usually single function.

Members are supported in their work by the executive staff based at the UKCC's offices at 23 Portland Place, London. The staff, headed by a chief executive/registrar, have a wide range of roles and responsibilities. A key area of activity is obviously associated with supporting the Council members in their policy and standards work, either in the formulation of new policies on a range of matters, such as education, professional conduct or aspects of professional practice, or in the revision of existing policies. This involves preparation of material, the marshalling and presentation of the relevant facts and contributing to the ensuring debates. Effectively servicing the Council meeting, the committees and task groups carry out complex and demanding work, both administratively and professionally.

Another area of regular Council activity that everyone will know about is the work associated with the Council's disciplinary functions, dealing with the 900 or so complaints of misconduct or unfitness to practice through ill health received each year from members of the public, professionals and employers. Professional conduct hearings take place most weeks of the year.

The registration department is the nerve centre of the organization's day-to-day work and is always busy, handling calls and visits from nurses, midwives and health visitors qualified both in the UK and overseas, who are seeking registration, changes to their registration or general information.

A few interesting statistics – did you know that the UKCC handles *each day* around 14 000 items of post, 2000 changes to the register, 5000 telephone calls (which you will know if you have ever tried to phone up!), and 1200 calls to the confirmations service.

The Council also offers a well-used professional advice service for more than 4000 person hours a year. Individual members of the profession ring the Council with a huge range of professional queries daily, many of them about PREP, but also, to name but a few, on issues to do with roles and responsibilities, professional accountability, confidentiality, difficult work relationships, advertising and poor clinical practice,

Work undertaken

To put some flesh on the bones of the above facts, it might be helpful just to look briefly at some of the work that the UKCC has undertaken since its inception (see Box 4.1)

Box 4.1   Some key UKCC milestones since its inception

1982   The first edition of *The Code of Professional Conduct* (UKCC 1982) is published

1983   Direct elections to the National Boards

1984   Second edition of *The Code of Professional Conduct* (UKCC 1984) is published

1985   Work starts on Project 2000
Advertising by Registered Nurses, Midwives and Health Visitors (UKCC 1985) is published

1986   Periodic registration is introduced
The first edition of the *Midwives Rules* (UKCC 1986a) and *The Midwife's Code of Practice* (UKCC 1986b) are published
The Project 2000 report *A New Preparation for Practice* (UKCC 1986c) is published
Administrations of Medicines (UKCC 1986d) published

1987   *Confidentiality* (UKCC 1987) published

1988   End of the first term of office of the Council, start of the second term
Project 2000 proposals accepted
Supplementary paper on Administration of Medicines (UKCC 1998) published

1989   PREPP starts
Exercising Accountability (UKCC 1989) published

1990   PREPP work continues

1991   *Report on Community Education and Practice* (UKCC 1991) published

1992   Third edition of *The Code of Professional Conduct* (UKCC 1992a) published
First edition of *The Scope of Professional Practice* (UKCC 1992b) published
First edition of *Standards for the Administration of Medicines* (UKCC 1992c) published
First edition of *A Guide for Students of Nursing and Midwifery* (UKCC 1992d) published
The Nurses, Midwives and Health Visitors Act 1992 (HMSO 1992)

1993   *Midwives Rules* (UKCC 1993a) published
Standards for Records and Record Keeping (UKCC 1993b) published
Complaints about Professional Conduct (UKCC 1993c) published

1994   *The Council's Standards for Post Registration Education and Practice* (the PREP report) (UKCC 1994a) published
Government approval secured for PREP proposals
The Midwives Code of Practice (UKCC 1994b) published
Professional Conduct – Occasional Report on Standards of Nursing Homes (UKCC 1994c) published
PREP fact sheets (UKCC 1994d) published

1995   PREP legislation came into force
The Council's Proposed Standards for Incorporation into Contracts for Hospital and Community Health Care Services (UKCC 1995a) published
Position Statement on Clinical Supervision for Nursing and Health Visiting (UKCC 1995b) published

1996   *Guidelines for Professional Practice* published (UKCC 1996a) (replacing *Exercising Accountability, Confidentiality, Advertising by Registered Nurses, Midwives and Health Visitors*)
Code of Best Practice for Members (UKCC 1996b) published
Issues Arising from Professional Conduct Complaints (UKCC 1996c) published
Reporting Misconduct – Information for Employers and Managers (UKCC 1996d) published
Reporting Unfitness to Practice (UKCC 1996e) published
Scope in Practice (UKCC 1996f) published

1997   *Handbook* (UKCC 1997a) published
Protecting the Public (UKCC 1997b) published
Enrolled Nursing – an Agenda for Action (UKCC 1997c) published
PREP and You (UKCC 1997d) published
Midwives Refresher course and PREP (UKCC 1997e) published

Relationships with other bodies

The primary legislation *requires* the Council to consult with 'representative of any group of persons who appear likely to be affected' when making new rules. There is therefore no choice in the matter. Indeed, one of the things that has to be confirmed before the drafting of any new rule gets underway is that consultation has taken place. However, the Council has increasingly, over its life span, sought to engage as many players as possible in its policy-making process. This started with Project 2000 but was expanded to a considerable extent during the PREP project.

Increasingly, the Council will involve some or all – depending on the issue under discussion – of the following groups and individuals in its debates:

- membership organizations
- National Boards
- employers
- purchasers/providers of education and health services
- individual registrants
- government departments in all four countries of the UK
- consumer organizations
- other health professions.

Contact can be made in a number of ways. With many organizations and groups, regular contact is already in place through regular meetings. There are also an increasing number of events around the UK where individuals have the opportunity to talk to Council members and officers about current and proposed issues. Council officers take every opportunity to go out and meet members of the professions in every possible circumstance, whether it be by speaking engagements to small or large groups, visits to clinical practice or in other ways.

Regular contacts with other groups and individuals is essential for the Council. It is one of the key ways in which it can ensure that its standards and policy work is relevant, responsive, cost-effective, patient/client-focused, implementable and measurable. It is also one of the means of ensuring that the efforts of all those bodies with an interest in furthering good, effective and compassionate nursing, midwifery and health visiting care – even if they come at the issues from different angles – can work together on the real issues affecting the professions.

REFERENCES

Committee on Nursing 1972 Report of the committee on nursing (Briggs report). HMSO (Cmnd 5115), London
Department of Health 1997 Press release 97/062 – review of the nurses, midwives and health visitors act. Richmond House, London
HMSO 1979 The Nurses, Midwives and Health Visitors Act 1979. HMSO, London

HMSO 1983 The Nurses Midwives and Health Visitors (Professional Conduct) Rules Approval Order 1983. Statutory Instrument 887. HMSO, London

HMSO 1992 The Nurses, Midwives and Health Visitors Act 1992. HMSO, London

HMSO 1995 The Nurses, Midwives and Health Visitors (Periodic Registration) Amendment Rules Approval Order 1995. Statutory Instrument 967. HMSO, London

The Stationery Office 1997 The Nurses, Midwives and Health Visitors Act 1997. The Stationery Office, London

UKCC 1982 Code of professional conduct. UKCC, London (out of print)

UKCC 1984 Code of professional conduct, 2nd edn. UKCC, London (out of print)

UKCC 1985 Advertising by registered nurses, midwives and health visitors. UKCC, London (out of print)

UKCC 1986a Midwives rules, 1st edn. UKCC, London (out of print)

UKCC 1986b The midwife's code of practice. UKCC, London

UKCC 1986c Project 2000: a new preparation for practice. UKCC, London

UKCC 1986d Administration of medicines. UKCC, London (out of print)

UKCC 1987 Confidentiality. UKCC, London (out of print)

UKCC 1988 Supplementary paper on administration of medicines. UKCC, London

UKCC 1989 Exercising accountability. UKCC, London (out of print)

UKCC 1991 Report on community education and practice. UKCC, London

UKCC 1992a Code of professional conduct, 3rd edn. UKCC, London

UKCC 1992b The scope of professional practice. UKCC, London

UKCC 1992c Standards for the administration of medicines. UKCC, London

UKCC 1992d A guide for students of nursing and midwifery. UKCC, London

UKCC 1993a Midwives rules. UKCC, London

UKCC 1993b Standards for records and record keeping. UKCC, London

UKCC 1993c Complaints about professional conduct. UKCC, London

UKCC 1994a The council's standards for post registration and practice (the PREP report). UKCC, London

UKCC 1994b Midwives code of practice. UKCC, London

UKCC 1994c Professional conduct – occasional report on standards in nursing homes. UKCC, London

UKCC 1994d PREP fact sheets. UKCC, London (out of print)

UKCC 1995a The council's proposed standards for incorporation into contracts for hospital and community health care services. UKCC, London

UKCC 1995b Position statement on clinical supervision for nursing and health visiting. UKCC, London

UKCC 1996a Guidelines for professional practice. UKCC, London

UKCC 1996b Code of best practice for members. UKCC, London

UKCC 1996c Issues arising from professional conduct complaints. UKCC, London

UKCC 1996d Reporting misconduct – information for employers and managers. UKCC, London

UKCC 1996e Reporting unfitness to practice. UKCC, London

UKCC 1996f Scope in practice. UKCC, London

UKCC 1997a Handbook. UKCC, London

UKCC 1997b Protecting the public. UKCC, London

UKCC 1997c Enrolled nursing – an agenda for action. UKCC, London

UKCC 1997d PREP and you. UKCC, London

UKCC 1997e Midwives refresher courses and PREP. UKCC, London

The PREP story

What's past is prologue

(*The Tempest*, William Shakespeare)

INTRODUCTION

This chapter looks at the setting up of the project that became known as PREPP (post-registration education and practice project) – the second of the UKCC's major projects to take place, since its establishment in 1983. It is not a story which has been told elsewhere and, as such, will be of interest to readers in a variety of ways. It describes how the UKCC planned and executed a major project in a manner which was designed specifically to involve all those who would be affected by its outcomes, either directly or indirectly, building on the interactive and consultative approach which it was already trying to make a hallmark of its work. As you know by now, if you didn't before, there are over 640 000 individuals registered with the UKCC and we will all be affected, to a greater or lesser extent, by the PREP requirements. So it should be helpful, in terms of having a better understanding of the origins of PREP and the work that underpinned its final decisions. As to whether PREP(P) has one 'P' or two, you will soon find the answer – please read on.

I am sure that many people, myself included before I went to work at the UKCC, have this rather vague notion of how policy is made in 'ivory towers'. So, for those of you who want to know the realities of the processes and practicalities of policy-making, it might make interesting reading.

Like so many issues of such strategic importance, its origins go back some way, and to an extent the building blocks were set out in the previous chapter. It is essential at this point, however, to remind ourselves of the reforms of pre-registration nursing and midwifery education which took place in the 1980s and became known as Project 2000.

PROJECT 2000

Although the purpose of this book is not to look in detail at Project 2000, it must be given its rightful place in the sequence of the development of the professions and the work of the UKCC, as it plays an essential part in the background to what became known as the PREP project.

In 1984 the UKCC set up a group 'to determine the education and training required in preparation for the professional practice of nursing, midwifery and health visiting in relation to the projected health needs in the 1990s and beyond and to make recommendations' (UKCC 1996). Thus was Project 2000 born. This was the first opportunity since the formation and full operation of the new statutory framework to carry out a wide-ranging review of educational preparation for nursing, midwifery and health visiting in all four countries of the UK. It was an operation designed to be carried out 'in the sunshine', involving as many interested parties as possible in the debates which were to take place.

As you will know, Project 2000 subsequently proposed wide-ranging and significant changes to pre-registration preparation for nurses and midwives, which after discussion and modification were finally accepted and implemented in all four countries of the UK. Some of the key Project 2000 recommendations related to:

- the establishment of one level of nurse
- the organization of the initial nursing preparation into an 18 month common foundation programme
- 18 month branch programmes, followed by registration in adult nursing, mental health nursing, mental handicap nursing (subsequently to be known as learning disabilities nursing) and children's nursing
- supernumerary status for students
- a new 'helper' grade, supervised by registered practitioners
- the continuation of the post-registration programme of 18 months for midwives and further development of 3 year midwifery programmes.

In addition, there were a number of significant recommendations which were to be relevant to the PREP project (the numbering is taken from *Project 2000: A New Preparation For Practice*; UKCC 1986, p. 70):

- Recommendation 10: there should be a coherent, comprehensive cost-effective framework of education beyond registration.
- Recommendation 11: there should be specialist practitioners, some of whom will also be team leaders, in all areas of practice in hospital and community settings. The requisite qualifications will be recordable on Council's register.
- Recommendation 12: health visiting, occupational health nursing and school nursing should be specialist qualifications which are recordable on the Council's register.
- Recommendation 13: district nursing, community psychiatric nursing and community mental handicap nursing should be specialist qualifications which are recordable on Council's register.

THE SETTING UP OF PREPP

A word of explanation about the acronyms would probably be helpful here. The work from 1989 to 1994 was project work. You will therefore see the acronym PREPP used, standing for 'Post Registration and Practice Project'. After 1994, when the proposals were accepted, the project came to an end. It is therefore at this stage that the final 'P' was dropped and PREP appears. This is actually still a shorthand – albeit a memorable one – for the 'UKCC's post-registration education and practice (PREP) requirements'. Interestingly, as is often the way with the evolution of language, the acronym has taken on its own lease of life and is now frequently used as a noun, as in 'doing my PREP' or 'what are you doing for your PREP this year?'.

The systems are put into place

The Council agreed to start work on the standard, kind and content of post-registration preparation in August 1988.This was at the end of the 1985–1989 Council term of office. Members were eager to get work underway before the next Council took up its term of office in November 1989, so that the broad strategic direction was already planned and there would be no loss of continuity in the proposed work. Some preliminary activity had already been undertaken, without significant conclusion, on return to practice programmes and periodic refreshment for nurses and health visitors. Midwives, of course, had already had statutory requirements in place in relation to refresher courses and return to practice requirements since the 1930s. A post-Project 2000 working group of UKCC and National Board members had also undertaken some more work on the concept of the specialist practitioner in 1986.

A paper went to the Council in November 1988 which identified three key aspects of post-registration activity that needed concentrated work. These were:

- formal post-registration activities
- periodic refreshment for nurse and health visitors
- re-entry programmes for nurses and health visitors who had been out of practice.

A special strategy conference in January 1989 discussed the matters further and Council, at its meeting in February 1989, agreed to remit the work to its Education Policy Advisory Committee (EPAC) to take forward. The outcome was a formal recommendation to the Council that an EPAC-led project be set up to establish 'a comprehensive current framework for standards relating to post-registration and practice'. EPAC further recommended that three working groups be established to look at:

- the nature of professional practice
- the processes of professional education and development
- requirements for continuing competence to practice.

It was considered important that full account be taken of the work previously done by the Council and National Boards, that meetings should be held with the National Boards and that the Boards be invited to appoint representatives to the three working groups. This was duly done.

The project was then formally established with Heather Williams, the Council's deputy registrar, as project director and myself as deputy director, concurrently with my role as assistant registrar, education and registration. I took over as director in 1993, at a time when the broad policy recommendations had been set out and work was starting on the standards for implementation. Professor Margaret Green, chairman of EPAC, was appointed chairman of the project steering group, which was to provide guidance and advice on the conduct of the project. A project office was established with an administrator and research assistant, together with a project team of the UKCC's professional officers who were to be very involved in helping with the work. The project fell into six fairly clearly defined chronological stages, which are used here as the framework to describe its progress. For ease of reference, the key stages are listed in Table 5.1.

Right from the start of the project, every effort was made to keep the nursing, midwifery and health visiting professions at large, and others with an interest in the work, informed of the project and its aims. At this stage a press briefing was held as were meetings with representatives of professional organizations and trade unions. In addition, every letter sent out to members of the professions from the Council contained a note letting them know about the project. A special meeting was held with the four National Boards and it was agreed that they would receive regular progress reports. The work already done by the Boards on the developments in continuing education were incorporated into the project's information systems.

Table 5.1 The key stages of the PREP project, 1989–1994

Year	Month	Event
1989	May	Council establishes project under EPAC (stage 1)
1990	January–March	Discussion document circulated to the professions for comment (stage 1)
1990	October	*The Report of the Post-registration Education and Practice Project* circulated for consultation (stage 2)
1990	November	Council appoints steering group to oversee further work on porject (stage 2)
1991	January	Council establishes Project on Community Education and Practice (CEP) under steering group (stage 3)
1991	July	Council receives a report on cost and benefit analysis of PREPP proposals (stage 2)
1991	July	Council receives analysis of responses to consultation on PREPP and agrees recommendations
		New steering group takes responsibility for overseeing the development of PREPP policy (stage 4)
1991	October	*Report on Proposals for the Future of Community Education and Practice* (CEP) circulated for comment (stage 3)
1992	February	Council agrees PREPP policy and establishes a new steering group to determine standards for post-registration education (stage 5)
1992	February	Council receives analysis of responses to CEP consultation and agrees that standards for community preparation be remitted to the above steering group (stage 5)
1993	March	*Consultation on the Council's Standards for Post Registration Education* circulated for comment (stage 5)
1993	October	Council receives analysis of responses to above document (stage 5)
1994	February	Council produces final report *The Future of Professional Practice – the Council's Standards for Education and Practice following Registration* (stage 6)

Stage 1: the work gets underway (August 1988–May 1990)

As the project had started with three clearly defined areas for consideration, three working groups were established to take the work forward to look at the nature of professional practice, the processes of professional education and development and the requirements for continuing competence to practise. The group consisted of members of the Council and National Boards, all nurses, midwives and health visitors, with relevant experience in professional practice and representing the four countries of the UK. A professional officer was assigned to service each group.

Right from the start, the group that generated maximum discussion and indeed, dissension, was that looking at what became known as the 'spheres of practice' – in other words, specialist and advanced practice. Another area that provoked a healthy debate was that of maintaining standards for practice following registration. The Council's initial (unpublished) work on mandatory periodic refreshment had proved very inconclusive, even though there was a firm commitment to the concept and principles of maintaining and developing professional knowledge and competence. It was at this stage that the idea of the use of the personal professional profile was first mooted.

There was only one special event held during this period and that was with the professors of nursing. Its purpose was to explore and discuss the nature of professional practice. It was an interesting event but, other than a fairly basic definition of nursing, no significant consensus was reached.

It became clear quite quickly, during this stage, that the issues being raised were merely the tip of a very large iceberg and that the discussions which were taking place were going to be the preliminary round of a much bigger and more complex exercise. In preparation for this, a discussion document was prepared which was to be distributed as widely as possible, to start to gather the views of the professions on the issues which had been identified.

The discussion document was circulated in January 1990. It went out to the National Boards, the professional organizations and health authorities, inviting a response to a series of questions. In addition, the document was sent to any groups or individuals who requested it. The spring 1990 edition of *Register* – the UKCC publication sent free to all those on the register – included an article on the issues under debate, together with a pre-paid card for replies.

At this stage, each health authority (as they were then constituted, with a role in service provision) was invited to appoint a 'link officer' who would act as a conduit of UKCC information on PREPP and also attend special invitation events designed to ensure that as much accurate information as possible was disseminated out into their own 'patches'. They were also informed of the roadshows and proved a useful resource in identifying suitable venues within their areas.

A total of 20 roadshows were held, one in each of the then regional health authorities in England and two each in Scotland, Wales and Northern Ireland. Each event consisted of what became a regularly utilized format – the morning event was for an invited audience of those who were in positions from which they could cascade the information down to as many staff as possible; and the afternoon event was a completely open event for whoever wished to attend. Approximately 100 people attended each morning session and 200 in the afternoon. Officers and members also undertook a wide range of speaking engagements, specifically to discuss the project. In addition, all staff made a point of referring to the project when undertaking other speaking engagements, so that as many of the profession as possible could be accurately informed of what was going on.

There were three ways of responding to the discussion document and some individuals took advantage of all three methods: individuals could respond to the discussion papers; they could complete the questionnaire in *Register*; or they could attend one of the roadshows. A total of 29 278 responses were analysed, excluding those from the National Boards, which were undertaken separately. The total number contributing to the discussion was 402 126.

The questions raised in the discussion document included the following issues:

- Should there be three spheres of professional practice, i.e. initial, specialist and advanced?
- Should post-registration educational activity attract academic accreditation together with professional validation?
- Should academic accreditation incorporate the concept of credit accumulation?
- Should there be a statutory requirement for practitioners to hold the necessary relevant professional qualifications before practising in (a) the specialist sphere and (b) the advanced sphere of practice?
- Should there be the introduction of a review system for all practitioners and if so, how should it be operated?
- What should go into the personal professional profile and should it be linked to any review system?

There was a lot of helpful comment and discussion on the issues raised. The key issues which needed clarification were identified and areas of concern noted. These are set out in detail in the next section.

One additional issue raised at this time was the way in which consultations of this complex and diverse nature should be carried out, specifically in terms of the weighting given variously to the responses from individuals and those from organizations representing a much larger number of people. It was agreed that expert advice should be sought on this issue. This is referred to again later in the chapter.

Stage 2: moving on (May 1990–July 1991)

This stage of the project started with a 2 day conference in Harrogate. Many of the meetings of the project group took place out of London. It was considered important to get everyone out of their familiar surroundings, so that there were no distractions and all minds could be focused on the matter in hand. The purpose of the conference was:

- to take note of the responses to the discussion document
- to discuss in detail the issues arising
- to plan a programme of work.

Proposals for post-registration education were to be finalized and incorporated into a draft report to be submitted to the Council by 3 July 1990. A number of key issues were identified in the document, which needed to be addressed.

One of the most important issues raised at this stage of the discussion by those responding was that of the support needed by newly qualified practitioners. Respondents felt that the 'transition' stage from student to registered practitioner was a very stressful period and that the existing ad hoc arrangements (if any) did not adequately support the newly qualified. A number of people felt that the supervision arrangements for health visitors and district nurses was a model worthy of consideration. This is where the idea of preceptorship was first raised, although at the time there was considerable debate over which term should be used to describe the concept of support for the newly qualified practitioner.

As had been the case in Project 2000 and would continue to be so in PREPP, the issue of the 'spheres' of professional practice aroused strong feelings and lively debate. The term 'initial', relating to the first phase of professional practice, was dropped in favour of 'primary', although that was also dispensed with, in due course. Although it was broadly considered that 'specialist' referred to working in a speciality and that 'advanced' was therefore more appropriate, no consensus could be reached on differences between specialist and advanced. It was therefore agreed that for the purposes of the report in hand, reference be made to 'specialist/advanced', in order to avoid slowing down the momentum of the project and to keep the work moving forward.

Maintaining and developing professional knowledge and competence were other issues needing detailed debate. The idea of profiling had been accepted by the profession even at this stage in the discussion but there was a range of issues raised about what should be included within the profile and the method of verification of its contents. The responses had also shown that the profession felt that it would be essential to make study leave a statutory requirement to ensure that it was undertaken.

As a policy decision had already been made to implement a statutory requirement for return to practice programmes, it was agreed that this be included in the final report, together with details as to what constituted a break in practice and the outcomes of return to practice programmes.

Other matters which were raised at this stage included:

- the position of enrolled nurses
- the position of health visitors
- credit accumulation and transfer
- eligibility to practice and registration.

Two other important issues were raised which also needed consideration, although they were not about the content of the proposed report. One issue related to the way in which responses to the previous consultation docu-

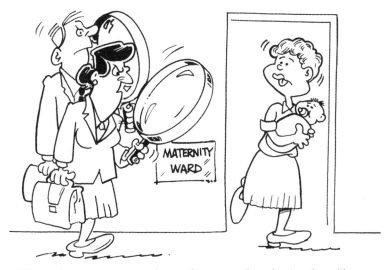

'The main worry expressed over the personal professional profile was over its verification.'

ments had been dealt with. Some dissatisfaction had been expressed at the way the responses had been presented, particularly over the weighting of the replies – for example, how do you compare the single response from an individual midwife with the single response from the Royal College of Midwives, representing several thousand practitioners. We went to see a statistician at the Social Science Research Council, who agreed that with so many divergent groups it was inappropriate to merely total the responses. He recommended that colour-coding be used to identify each main group responding, e.g. health authorities, and that the replies be analysed separately. In that way it would be possible to see how each group responded to each question and members could form their own views on the weight to give to each reply, as they had all the information in front of them. From then on, this was how the responses to consultation were presented.

There was also the issue of who should write the report. It was thought to be very important that the report was written by someone who could move away from 'Council speak' and produce a document that set the issues out clearly but also in a style which was friendly and readable. We were lucky enough to get the services of Tim Rice, then working as a journalist for *The Times* newspaper. He had previously been on the staff of the *Nursing Times*, and so was familiar with many of the issues under discussion. From then on he worked closely with officers to produce the report.

The agreed report, *The Report of the Post-registration and Practice Project* (UKCC 1990), was circulated for consultation in October 1990. There was to be a 6 month period of consultation. It was sent to specific organizations and a copy given to individuals on request. In addition, every practitioner on the register was sent an extended summary of the report with a page for responses. The Council itself and the National Boards had had an opportunity to comment in July 1990.

Whilst the consultation was taking place, more activity was going on to progress other important aspects of the work. In January 1991, the Council set up a complementary project on community education and practice – an area that had been identified as urgently needing more detailed attention. This is described more fully in the next section on stage 3.

In November 1990, a new steering group was established on post-registration and practice, which would report directly to the Council, unlike the previous work which had been done as part of the remit of the Education Policy Advisory Group. The chair of the new group was Margaret Green and Heather Williams, and I remained as director and deputy director. The group's purpose was to carry forward the policy work arising from the PREPP proposals.

A cost–benefit analysis was undertaken by the management consultants Price Waterhouse during this phase of the work. They obtained a lot of their information from a panel selected from the link officers with health authorities and, in addition, they undertook a number of special field trips out to authorities who were known to have undertaken costing of post-registration education activity. It is interesting with the benefit of hindsight to note that at this stage, very few organizations were able to give a clear account of their sources of post-registration funding. However, a very detailed report on the Price Waterhouse findings was subsequently made to the Council in March 1991 with an amended summary in July 1991. The estimated costs to implement all the PREPP proposals were £15–30 million (this broad range reflecting the absence or inconsistency of the information at the authorities visited on field trips or otherwise consulted) and the continuing costs were stated as being £129–£169 per year for all practitioners. The results of the consultation, meanwhile, were being received and then analysed. They were presented to the Council in July 1991. A total of 35 999 documents were received, with 33 667 being the responses to the *Register* questionnaire. The overall response was positive. The main concerns that were identified were:

- the costs and manpower implications
- the need for guidelines
- the need for further consultation on the standard, kind and content of advanced practice
- clarification of the verification of the personal professional profile.

The proposed recommendations and the Council's response are detailed on pages 87–90.

Stage 3: community education and practice (July 1990–March 1992)

Whilst the above activity was being undertaken, the Council was concurrently running a separate but related project on community education and practice. To make sense of it, we need to go back a little in time to July 1990. This was when the Council had considered a paper which set out the implications of the NHS and Community Care Act 1990 (HMSO 1990) which, together with reforms of pre-registration nursing education, had implications for community practice and education. As a consequence of this and other discussions, it was agreed to hold a major 'summit' meeting on 30 November–1 December 1990, in order to:

- identify the key issues that need to be addressed to provide an effective community service and
- to formulate a strategy to resolve problems in the current provision of community education, both in the short and the long term.

The summit was attended by general secretaries of the relevant professional organizations/trade unions, the chief nursing officers of the four government health departments and the chairmen and chief officers of the four National Boards. It was agreed that a project group should be set up to explore further the issues raised. This group would be a subgroup of the Steering Group on Post-Registration Education and Practice. Two key statements were agreed as a basis for the work, which were agreed by all those present. First that the term 'primary health care nursing' was acceptable but it needed to be developed and expanded. Second, there was *no* support for the idea that there should be direct entry into primary health care nursing – in other words, preparation for primary health care nursing should always follow an initial nursing qualification. It was further agreed that the idea of primary health care nursing needed to be explored against the concepts of primary, specialist and advanced practice as previously described in the PREP report.

The Council agreed the proposals at its meeting in January 1991 and Kay Rogers, a health visitor Council member, was appointed chairman of the subgroup. The project group appointed had a membership which was broadly representative of all community nursing interests. The project was managed by the PREPP director and deputy director. It was required to report back to Council by May 1991. In the 5 months it had to complete its work, the project group met with, amongst others, the Council's Midwifery Committee and the Health Visiting and District Nursing Joint Committee. The main discussions centred around:

- whether the term primary health nursing or community health care nursing, to link with the Community Care Act, was more appropriate

- the identification of the educational requirements for community health care
- links between these requirements and the framework for post-registration education and practice
- what differences in preparation would be needed for community practice by those who had done a Project 2000 programme and those who had not
- how the models of primary, specialist and advanced could be applied to community practice.

An interim report was produced for the Council in May 1991 and it was further agreed to have a second summit meeting in June 1991 to brief participants on progress. The outcomes of all these deliberations was a report entitled *Report on Proposals for the Future of Community Education and Practice* which went out to the profession and relevant organizations for consultation on 1 October 1991, with a 3 month consultation period.

The consultation document did not contain specific recommendations and did not have a specific response sheet. The issues for debate and consideration were, however, set out clearly in sections, as follows:

- community health care nursing
- the position of nursing, midwifery and health visiting
- the issues
- health care needs
- the discipline of community health care nursing
- future preparation
- the position of existing practitioners.

A total of 1165 documents were received in response and the total number contributing was 6650.The overall responses to the proposals were favourable and everyone agreed that action on future preparation needed to be addressed as a matter of urgency. The majority of those responding wanted more detail on the standard, kind and content of preparation for practice in the community and were clearly expecting further consultation at some stage.

There were three main areas of concern. First, many respondents were worried that the Council was, in effect, proposing a generic community heath care nurse. A lot of opposition was expressed to this idea. Second, there had been no specific identification of the community paediatric nurse and no mention had been made of the care of the sick child in the community. This was felt to be a major omission. Third, there were concerns expressed by those already working in the community as to how their knowledge and experience would be recognized. Some thought that their existing qualifications would not be recognized and that they would have to undertake further training. There were also concerns expressed by those who were working in the community but who had no formal community qualifications. Many felt that they should be given recognition on the basis of their considerable experience. The group expressing the greatest concern on this issue were practice nurses.

Having considered these responses the Council made a number of policy decisions. It agreed the following:

- The term 'community health care nurse' was to be used, with clarification that a 'generic' practitioner was *not* being proposed.
- Specialist preparation would be required for specific areas of practice to meet the needs of the community.
- Practitioners already working with a recognized community qualification which was registrable or recordable would be automatically recognized as a community health care nurse.
- Other nurses would be required to do additional preparation and credit could be obtained for relevant experience and qualifications.
- Enrolled nurses would need to complete additional preparation which would also incorporate conversion to a first level qualification.
- The standard, kind and content of educational preparation for nurses would be considered by the steering group already set up by the Council to look at the education that would lead to additional qualifications at post-registration level.

It was anticipated that the steering group would have completed its work before the Autumn of 1992, so that new education programmes could begin in 1993.

Stage 4: policy development (July 1991–February 1992)

And so, back to the main project. The Council decided on a programme of implementation for each of its key PREPP recommendations, set out below, after having considered the responses to the consultation at its meeting in July 1991. These decisions were made known to the professions in a press statement. They dealt with the following aspects of the post-registration framework.

Support and preceptorship

Recommendations 1 and 2: a period of support should be provided for newly qualified practitioners by preceptors at the time of each new registration.

It was agreed that, as this idea had already been fully supported, guidance should be issued shortly on its implementation. It was further agreed that the recommendations were not to be a statutory requirement, but to be guidance on good practice. Concern had been expressed over the position of those individuals who had been unable to find employment on registration, those working independently, and those working for agencies. It was agreed that these issues should be addressed in the guidance, and that an exploratory study be undertaken to monitor newly registered practitioners over a period of a year, in order to obtain information on the degree of support given and the use of preceptors, once the recommendations had been made public.

Personal professional profile

Recommendations 3, 4 and 5: all practitioners must demonstrate that they have maintained and developed their professional knowledge and competence; a personal professional profile should be completed as a record of experience and achievements as they develop their practice and a minimum of 5 days of study leave every 3 years should be allowed to each practitioner.

The main worry expressed over the personal professional profile was in relation to its verification. It had originally been suggested that verification be undertaken by another practitioner, but there was growing concern that this may be used inappropriately. After considerable discussion, it was agreed that the most appropriate form of verification would be self-verification. This would reaffirm the UKCC's commitment to the trust it placed in its registrants. It was also agreed that a paper be taken to the Council in November 1991, to look at profiling and audit systems.

The subsequent work agreed that practitioners should keep their profiles in a form that could be given to the Council, at its request, as documentary evidence that its requirements had been met. It was further agreed, at this stage, that the Council would meet the cost of providing every practitioner with a binder in which to keep the profile. It could not be a statutory requirement that the Council folder be used, but it was felt that, as the concept of profiling was still comparatively new, this would help to provide a general standard. The actual cost of providing profiles was estimated at being between £1 million and £4 million for the first 3 years and approximately £1 million thereafter, depending upon the number of newly registered practitioners.

This decision was subsequently rescinded in May 1994 because there were by then so many profiles available on the market, of all ranges, cost and quality, that it was agreed it would not be a good use of practitioners' money to spend it on providing Council profiles. Instead it was decided to provide detailed guidance to every practitioner about completing a profile and the nature of its contents.

Return to practice programmes

Recommendation 6: those wishing to return to practice after a break of 5 years or more must complete a return to practice programme.

The need for these programmes to be made statutory for nurses and health visitors after a break of 5 years or more was fully supported. There was, however, concern expressed about cost. It was agreed to provide information on the standard, kind and content of programmes for the Council to consider at its meeting in November 1991. It was agreed that the requirement should be implemented as soon as possible, as good practice, and that it become a statutory requirement from 1993, once the legislation was in place. Midwives were to continue with their existing statutory requirements, including the annual notification of intention to practice, until the new PREP legislation, which was to include midwives, was in place. Once the new legislation was in place, the notification of intention to practice was also to be retained.

Advanced practice

Recommendation 7: in order to practise as an advanced practitioner in the fields of clinical expertise, education, research and management, advanced practitioners must have recorded a Council-approved recordable qualification.

Yet again there was no agreement on the preparation for advanced practice, as the concepts of primary, advanced and consultant practice were not fully understood. It was agreed that this needed further consideration and that the idea of specialist practice should be revisited. Discussions over the next few months looked at these issues in more detail and finally the idea of primary practice for nurses, midwives and health visitors, specialist for nurses and health visitors, and enhanced for midwives and advanced practice for all were agreed. Midwives rejected the concept of specialist practice for midwifery, as it was agreed that it was not appropriate to sub-divide midwifery into specialisms. The term 'enhanced' was therefore adopted for midwifery, as better fitting the concept of expanding the whole range of a midwife's knowledge and skills. The use of the term 'primary' was also debated at length, particularly in relation to any possible confusion with primary nursing. No decision to change it was made at this stage, however.

Eligibility to practise

Recommendations 8 and 9: registration with the UKCC will embrace a new concept of eligibility to practise which will demonstrate that practitioners have maintained and developed their professional knowledge and competence and identify their areas of practice.

The profession fully supported the new concept of 'eligibility to practise' for nurses and health visitors. That is, that the idea that registration should change significantly to become, in effect, a licence to practise. It was agreed that further information would be needed on how the notification of practice form would be implemented. Midwives were to continue with the statutorily required notification of intention to practice on an annual basis.

In February 1992, the Council agreed that the general policy on all the recommendations was now complete and that work should start on how the recommendations were to be implemented, using the register as the means of securing standards, with the exception of the standard, kind and content of post-registration education, on which further work needed to be done.

Stage 5: establishing standards for post-registration education (March 1992–October 1993)

Having broadly agreed the standards for maintaining registration the Council now turned to the new criteria for using the register in recording post-registration qualifications. Following a decision at the Council meeting in March 1992, a new steering committee was established, to undertake the work, chaired by Professor Margaret Green and with myself as project director. Five working groups were set up to look specifically at:

- issues for nursing practice
- issues for midwifery practice
- issues for community practice
- credit accumulation
- modularization and assessment.

Meetings took place at all times of day and night, in order to get the work done and to get a report to the Council by the autumn of 1992. Following the presentation of the draft report to the Council in October 1992, a series of seminars and meetings were held prior to the presentation of the final report to Council in March 1993. The report was agreed at the Council meeting. As a result, a further consultation document was prepared for the professions – *Consultation on the Council's Standards for Post-registration Education* (UKCC 1993a). There was a 5 month period of consultation from May 1993 until September 1993. The key issues related to the model of practice, a standards framework, existing practitioners, implementation, and standards for the teaching of nursing and midwifery. Let us look at these in turn.

The model of practice

In February 1992, the Council had agreed the terms for practice – 'primary' for nurses and midwives, 'specialist' for nurses, 'enhanced' for midwives, and 'advanced' for nurses and midwives. The terms had, however, remained the subject of intense debate and discussion. Members wanted to make it clear that the majority of practitioners would spend their professional careers working competently in primary practice – specialist practice would be for a comparatively small number of practitioners. It certainly was not envisaged that all practitioners would have, need or want a specialist qualification.

Enhanced practice, which had been applied to midwifery, was still felt by many to be inappropriate. The term 'expert' was explored and briefly adopted, but then abandoned again reluctantly in favour of 'enhanced'.

Advanced practice, as always, provoked much discussion. The main concern was that as it was felt that innovations in practice occur at all levels of practice, it would be inappropriate to label a specific element advanced. It was finally decided to have a special section on innovations in practice to make this explicit. It was also agreed that there needed to be a section on the nurse practitioner and to address how that role fitted into the model being proposed.

A standards framework

A lot of work had been done on trying to bring some coherence to the concept of 'specialist' and all the existing courses had been examined. It was finally agreed that a broad classification could be:

- critical care
- acute care
- continuing care.

The areas of speciality were listed under each section in the final report. Work done on the community preparation for nurses identified three main areas of skills activity which characterized specialist practice. It was subsequently agreed that these areas also applied to all specialist practice, not just the community. The three areas were clinical care, care and programme management, and team leadership. Team leadership was subsequently incorporated into care and programme management.

Existing practitioners and implementation

There was considerable discussion as to whether health visiting should continue to be registered in the future or whether some alternative system should be introduced. It was finally agreed that health visiting should continue as registrable qualification (to do otherwise would have required amendment of the primary legislation), but that specialist, enhanced and advanced qualifications would be recordable.

Standards for the teaching of nursing or midwifery

These are dealt with in a separate section on pages 93–96.

A total of 437 documents were received in response to the consultation document (UKCC 1993a), from employing authorities, educational institutions, membership organizations, National Boards, and medical and consumer organizations. In the main, the responses were positive and extremely helpful. However, it was felt that, overall, the whole framework was too hierarchical and rigid and needed much more flexibility, if it was to be sufficiently adaptable to meet changing service and individual practitioner needs. The specific issues raised as needing more clarification and attention were:

- grading implications in respect of employment
- time-scale for completion of the programme of implementation
- time-scale for the completion of the programmes of education
- enhanced midwifery practice
- budgetary and human resource implications.

Having considered both the qualitative and quantitative analysis of the responses to the consultation, the Council, at its meeting in October 1993, decided that the areas that needed revisiting (that were within the remit of the UKCC), to address the expressed concerns, were:

- the model of practice
- enhanced and advanced midwifery practice
- description of specialist practice
- areas of specialist practice and outcomes
- common core outcomes – community health care nursing.

It was agreed that the outcomes of this further work would be considered at a special seminar in January 1994 and for final agreement in February 1994 at the Council meeting.

Stage 6: the future of professional practice – the Council's standards for education and practice following registration (October 1993–May 1994)

This was the final stage of the actual PREPP project. Having considered the responses to the consultation paper in October 1993, further work had been done on the areas of concern and the Council was pleased to agree its final report on PREP in March 1994. As you can imagine, this decision was greeted with great delight and relief by all those who had been involved with the project.

The decisions which had been taken in response to the concerns raised during the consultation were to:

- Discard use of the term 'primary nursing' because of the identified confusion that might exist between that and primary nursing. Instead it was decided to refer to 'professional practice' to describe the area in which most nurses and midwives would spend the majority of their careers.
- Define specialist nursing practice and the explicit links between the possession of a specialist qualification, the Council's standards and the register.

- Discard the use of 'enhanced' in relation to midwifery, and describe the continuing nature of post-registration midwifery education, which is not linked to the explicit acquisition of specific qualifications for additional roles.
- Make it clear that no formal preparation and qualification with explicit links with the Council's register was being proposed, at this stage, for advanced practice. In addition, a general statement supporting the reality of advancing practice in all settings was to be made.
- Emphasize, in community health care nursing, the need for common core preparation for community nursing practice together with specialist modules relating to areas of practice. A period of supervised practice was also proposed.
- Enable enrolled nurses to achieve first level registration together with a specialist qualification, providing that they had met the outcomes for both programmes.
- Avoid specifying the number and type of specialist qualifications, outside the community, at this stage, but to allow programmes to evolve in response to service need.

Between March and May 1994, discussions were held with colleagues representing the four government departments. The Council was pleased to hear in May 1994 that government support had been secured for the final proposals. Although the UKCC is an independent body, financed by registrant's fees, government support is necessary on matters of significant policy change affecting large numbers of the professional workforce, especially where changes to the legislation need to be made. As the whole of the PREPP debate had been conducted with maximum publicity, with all relevant parties involved throughout, there were, of course, no major surprises in the final proposals. The consultative nature of the exercise also meant that the UKCC could genuinely say that its proposals had secured the support of the professions – indeed, significant changes had been made in response to consultation.

The next substantial activity was the implementation of the proposals and it was agreed that a paper be prepared for the Council meeting in July1994.

TEACHERS OF NURSING, MIDWIFERY AND HEALTH VISITING

The section sets out the history of the debate and decisions in relation to the recording of teaching qualifications for those teaching nursing, midwifery and health visiting. The wording is important as the issue was often misunderstood. What the UKCC was doing, as had the previous statutory and training bodies, was to consider what standards should apply to those who were teaching the subjects of nursing, midwifery and health visiting – *not* the standards for those who were teaching other subjects to individual nurses, midwives and health visitors.

In 1984, the then Education Policy Advisory Committee considered the different criteria which had been used by the previous statutory and training bodies and agreed that the Council needed to produce and publish clear criteria for those eligible to take posts as teachers of nursing, midwifery, district nursing, occupational health nursing and health visiting. The professions were consulted and the criteria were agreed. They related to the acquisition of:

- *Registration on an appropriate part of the UKCC register.* This was to ensure that the individual had the basic knowledge necessary of the area of professional practice that was being taught.
- *Relevant professional experience.* This was to ensure that those teaching the subject(s) had had the opportunity to consolidate their knowledge through a substantial period of professional practice, in order to provide a credible role model for students, in a practice-based profession.
- *Additional professional knowledge.* This was to ensure that those who were teaching had a wider and deeper knowledge of the subject than that acquired during initial preparation, in addition to that acquired through practice.
- *An appropriate teaching qualification.* Nursing, midwifery and health visiting had, for many years, required that those teaching in the professions were not only experienced in their own professional knowledge and practice, but were also able to impart their knowledge, by the acquisition of a teaching qualification. In this respect the professions regulated by the Council were many years in advance of the other health care professions, and indeed higher education itself, where knowledge of the subject was considered to be the only criteria for teaching it.

The criteria were subject to incremental modification over the years and it was agreed that the matter would be reconsidered within the framework for post-registration education and practice. The matter also needed urgent review, as nursing, midwifery and health visiting education had by this time moved, or was moving, into higher education, following the implementation of Project 2000.

The final report addressed the standards for teaching in the following way. It reiterated the fact that as nursing, midwifery and community health care nursing are practice-based professions, then it follows that those who are educating the practitioners in nursing, midwifery and community care nursing education and practice must themselves be both clinically credible and knowledgeable about contemporary practice. It was also recognized that a wide variety of experts, from a number of other disciplines, would also contribute to the teaching of students.

It was therefore agreed that to become a teacher of nursing, midwifery or community health care nursing, the practitioner must:

- be a graduate, with a specialist qualification recorded on the register, or with evidence of additional midwifery studies
- possess an appropriate teaching qualification, approved by a National Board, which is either at graduate or postgraduate level and incorporates supervised teaching practice
- possess relevant and up-to-date clinical experience
- possess up-to-date research-based clinical expertise
- possess the ability to teach effectively through a variety of methods.

In addition, it was agreed 'that any student undertaking a programme leading to a registrable or recordable qualification must be supervised clinically by someone who already has that qualification or who has the appropriate clinical or practical teaching experience.' (UKCC 1994)

Although initially there was relief that the report had addressed what was becoming the increasingly urgent issue of 'teachers', during 1994–95 there were an increasing number of misunderstandings about what the UKCC was really saying on the issue. The main concern was expressed by those in the community who felt that the position of the community practice teacher (CPT) was under threat. It was clear that further work needed to be done to resolve this issue as it was beginning to affect the take-up and provision of places on CPT courses. A working group of Council and National Boards officers and members met during 1995 and came up with a set of proposals that involved both broad standards framework and the details of implementation. However, when these proposals were put before the Council early in 1996 it felt unable to accept them, as the issue of practice-based teaching had still not been addressed to its satisfaction and they asked that further work be done.

In order to avoid any potential bias on what had become a somewhat contentious issue, with a number of increasingly entrenched positions being adopted by some of the players, it was agreed that the additional work be undertaken by an outside consultant. The consultant reported to the Joint Education Committee of the UKCC. A substantial consultation on a set of proposed standards was undertaken, which included a postal questionnaire and a series of meetings with respondents, in order to ensure that as many people as possible had a chance to make their views known. The main issues raised by respondents to the consultation were:

- the standards themselves, which were seen variously to be offering either too much or too little guidance (!)
- the amount of detail needed, on which there was little consensus
- the supervision of clinical/practice placements
- the differences between the different teaching roles, which were not sufficiently well described, particularly the different needs of pre- and post-registration students

- the need for teachers to be up-to-date with both education and practice issues, particularly the changes in health care delivery
- the need for teachers to have substantial practice experience
- the need for teachers to be graduates; while this was supported, concern was expressed over the possibility that a teaching qualification be acquired at the same time as a first degree
- teaching practice must be undertaken in a range of settings
- APEL mechanisms.

Following consultation and discussion of the results with the Joint Education and Midwifery Committees, further work was done on the draft standards. They were standards configured into four main areas to reflect the four key teaching roles identified during the consultation processes: those for mentor (i.e. with students), preceptor (already agreed by the UKCC as part of the original PREP standards), practice educator and lecturer. Outcomes were broadly grouped into those relating to:

- communications/relationships
- facilitate learning
- assessment
- role model*
- environment for Learning
- change*
- knowledge base
- course development.

(The two marked by asterisks are replaced by 'evaluation' and 'context of education' for lecturers.)

Although the UKCC agreed the proposals at its meeting in June 1997, further work still needed to be undertaken and was in progress at the time of this book going to print.

IMPLEMENTATION – 1994 ONWARDS

As you would expect, there was a huge amount of work to do once the standards had been agreed, and from 1994 through to 1996 regular activity was taking place in order to effectively implement PREP and to commence the monitoring and evaluation of the policies. The main activities are described below. Many of you reading this will have your own memories – partial and distorted though memories often are – of this time, as the PREP requirements actually started to 'hit the streets' and people began to realize that this 'thing' that had undergone such a long gestation was actually about to become a reality. I'm sure that there were lots of cynics – for whom I have a deal of sympathy – who thought it would never really happen.

Preparing and securing the legislation

Work started immediately the standards were finalized on putting the necessary legislation into place, as it had been agreed that the implementation date would be 1 April 1995. This would have been a tight time-frame for any new rules given the amount of work necessary for their preparation, let alone those of such far-reaching significance as the PREP requirements. The preparation of new rules is a complex business at the best of times, but this was particularly so with what became known as the 'PREP rules', as their preparation required an exploration of every aspect of the Council's existing legislation, to ensure that coherence and integrity were maintained throughout the whole of the Council's secondary legislation (the rules). It was necessary to consider in detail the effect of the proposed changes – particularly in relation to the standards for maintaining registration – on the existing rules relating to the UKCC's professional conduct procedures and the mechanical aspects of the registration process. A considerable amount of preparatory work was undertaken, in house, with the Council's officers and solicitor, ensuring that the intent of the policy was being accurately and appropriately translated into the draft rules. Once this initial stage was underway, detailed and lengthy discussions started with civil servant colleagues from the Department of Health in England, representing the four government health departments, and their solicitor, who provided advice on the actual drafting. This work continued throughout 1994 and into the early part of 1995 and consumed large amounts of time – at varying times of day and night, in order to meet the deadline.

The rules which permitted the implementation of the aspects of PREP relating to the maintenance and development of professional knowledge and competence came into force on 1 April 1995. The preparation had taken us right up to the deadline and the final version of the rules was signed and sealed by the UKCC's president and registrar/chief executive on 23 March 1995 and then signed by Virginia Bottomley as Secretary of State for Health on 30 March 1995 – so there was not much slack between signing and implementation on 1 April 1995! You can imagine that there was considerable rejoicing at having got such a complex and significant piece of legislation through, particularly in the agreed time-frame. For those who like to work from original sources, the 'PREP rules' are enshrined in Statutory Instrument (SI) 1995 No. 967 The Nurses, Midwives and Health Visitors (Periodic Registration) Amendment Rules Approval Order 1995 (HMSO 1995).

Review of policy on support and preceptorship

Another piece of work which was undertaken in 1994 was a review of the position in relation to the UKCC's requirements for a period of support, under the guidance of a preceptor. This position had been made public, as a statement of guidance on good practice in January 1993 (Registrar's Letter 1/1993 – the details of which are given in the next chapter; UKCC 1993b). A questionnaire survey was used to evaluate the implementation and interpretation of the policy. Additional guidance was issued in January 1995 (UKCC 1995b) to revise the original advice in order to correct some misunderstandings in relation to the policy and to ensure that it was implemented in a flexible and facilitative manner. Attention was drawn to the confusion which existed over the use of varying terms such as mentor, preceptor and clinical supervision. Particular attention was drawn to the initiatives on clinical supervision. The UKCC's position on support and preceptorship was felt to be entirely congruent with that on clinical supervision.

The registrar's letter states:

The Council believes that clinical supervision should cover the whole clinical career of a practitioner and this includes, therefore, the period of support and preceptorship offered to practitioners when they commence their careers. The statutory arrangements for the Supervision of Midwives and recent approaches to clinical supervision for nurse and health visitors are part of that continuum....

The other key message in the letter was to make it clear that the period of support was not being put into place as an extension of the programme of preparation leading to registration. The accountability of practitioners from the moment of registration was stressed. The main idea behind the period of support is to offer registered practitioners guidance from a more experienced colleague during the early months of professional practice, where individuals are competent but may not yet be very confident in their newly acquired knowledge and skills.

Preparation of information for registrants

PREP fact sheets

One of the most interesting activities during this period was the preparation of the information to the professions on the PREP requirements. In addition to the more traditional UKCC approach of registrar's letters and position statements – which are undoubtedly a vital and informative source of advice, albeit not written in a style necessarily designed to enthuse and enliven – it was agreed that something new should also be tried in order to convey the message about something as significant a change as PREP. This came about particularly after the UKCC agreed in March 1994 not to go ahead with the provision of personal professional profiles for all registrants, but rather to provide information for all those on the register on all elements of the requirements. A small working group consisting of four Council members, myself and the communications manager was set up to look at the issue and it was decided to call in the help of external design experts. The intention was to produce something in a format totally different from anything previously produced by the UKCC and which would immediately and visibly identify itself as the start of a new era in UKCC communications. This objective was certainly achieved. The PREP fact sheets were widely acclaimed as a breakthrough in the UKCC's style of communication. They were considered to be lively, informative and eye-catching, and an ideal start for the contents of an individual's personal professional profile. Every individual with an up-to-date registration with the UKCC was sent a personal copy in March 1995, with an accompanying letter from the UKCC president. In addition, unlimited numbers of the fact sheets were made available to registrants and other interested parties between April 1995 and December 1997, when they were replaced – on the grounds of both cost, convenience and expediency – by the useful UKCC booklet *PREP and you* (UKCC 1997).

UKCC/National Board conferences

More new ground was broken on the communications front during this period, by the organization of joint UKCC/National Board conferences, to disseminate information on the implementation of the PREP requirements. Conferences were organized throughout various locations in the UK, with four in England and two each in Scotland, Northern Ireland and Wales. A variety of interesting and unusual venues were chosen, including Leeds United Football Club. The conferences were well attended at both morning and afternoon sessions. Brief plenary sessions were used to introduce key themes and then workshops took place on the aspects of PREP which practitioners had identified as being of greatest interest and/or concern to them. Delegates could choose two out of four workshops, which covered profiling, maintaining registration, specialist practice and study activity. Presentations were made by officers from the UKCC and the National Boards, supported on many occasions by Council and Board members. The emphasis was on the translation of policy into reality – and how the statutory bodies could help the individuals concerned. It was also a good opportunity to look at how the national policy position was being implemented in each country of the UK. The demand for the conferences was so great that they were repeated again in England during 1996 – again taking place in four different locations throughout the country.

PREP helpline

One of the single most important actions during this period was the establishment of the PREP helpline. It was clear that a friendly and reliable source of information was needed to which practitioners could refer, on a regular basis, as they came to terms with the realities of PREP. The PREP helpline came into operation on 1 April 1995 and the phone has not stopped ringing

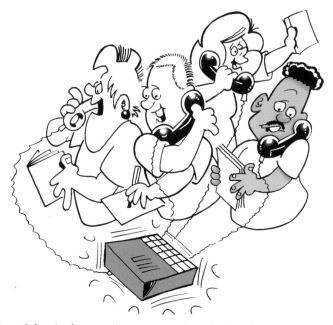

'One of the single most important actions during this period was the establishment of the PREP helpline.'

since! During the first year of operation, over 10 000 enquiries were dealt with, by letter and phone. The areas of greatest interest included who needed to maintain registration, the type of study activity that had to be undertaken, the use of personal professional profiles, how profiles would be audited, return to practice requirements, the requirements for specialist practice, CATS and APEL and the availability of appropriate courses.

The helpline was amalgamated with the professional advice service at the end of 1996, but a large number of the enquiries to the advice line continue to be on PREP. This is hardly surprising, as practitioners are rightly concerned about requirements that affect their registration and right to practise and need to be sure that they have accurate information on their own particular situation. Queries are also received in other parts of the UKCC, particularly in the registration department, where enquiries about the notification of practice form are especially numerous.

Other UKCC activity

During this time, a range of articles were produced by myself and other Council officers for the professional press on different aspects of the requirements. The Council's publication *Register* was also used to disseminate information. Indeed, the articles in *Register* became so popular that they became a regular feature of the middle spread – so that they could be easily detached and inserted into a professional profile. A section on common PREP questions and answers also proved popular, helping practitioners to realize that most people shared the same concerns. A whole range of speaking engagements was undertaken during this time with a wide variety of audiences, using every opportunity to spread the PREP message. As the successful implementation of PREP continued to fall within my personal objectives, during this period, I spent a lot of time on the road! I averaged about seven to 10 speaking engagements a month on the subject, during 1994–1996. In addition, other Council officers also made sure that PREP was addressed during their outside engagements, even if it wasn't the main item on the agenda. This was particularly the case for midwifery, as midwives needed clear and up-to-date information on how the new PREP requirements linked into their existing legislative requirements, in relation to refresher courses, return to practice requirements and notification of intention to practise.

One of the aspects of the work that I found very rewarding at this time was the interest expressed in the UKCC's activity by other professions, both within health care and more widely. Our standards were discussed, at their request, with – among others – representatives of general practitioners, hospital doctors, health service managers, dentists, pharmacists, engineers and lecturers in higher education. All those involved were, I believe rightly, impressed with the progress that we had made, particularly as it was for such large numbers of practitioners. In addition to the speaking engagements, the UKCC standards frequently featured in the data collected by a number of researchers who were looking at the systems being put into place for continuing professional development (CPD) amongst the professions. At a time when CPD initiatives were high on the agendas of many professions, the standards being set by the UKCC were seen as being in the vanguard for change and innovation.

Press and membership organization activity

In addition to the work already described, a range of articles appeared on different aspects of the requirements in the professional press and in the publications of the professional organizations. The professional organizations/trade unions were very helpful in spreading the message and some excellent additional advice was prepared by such organizations for their members. The professional press also threw themselves wholeheartedly into the provision of information on PREP, with both coverage of the UKCC activity and information on different aspects of the requirements, prepared by a variety of authors. Many organizations started to produce a range of material to support practitioners in meeting the UKCC's requirements, and a variety of interesting and imaginative media were used, particularly in the provision of study material. This activity has continued unabated and has considerably enhanced the individual professional's knowledge of, and interest in, PREP.

Specialist qualifications and transitional arrangements

The requirements for specialist qualifications had been made public in *The Future of Professional Practice – the Council's Standards for Education and Practice following Registration* (UKCC 1994) and subsequently, amongst other documents, in position statements 1 and 2 issued by the UKCC in March 1994 and March 1995 (UKCC 1994, 1995a). The standards for specialist qualifications were subject to review as implementation occurred, particularly as the UKCC wished to ensure that existing practitioners were offered as much support as possible if they wished to acquire additional qualifications.

One of the key issues that was particularly relevant at the time that the PREP proposals were being debated was that existing registered practitioners, particularly nurses, were already beginning to feel rather threatened by the 'new' breed of nurse that Project 2000 was by then starting to produce. There was a lot of concern and, to an extent, misinformation around and, understandably, people started to worry. Rumours were taking hold – quite inaccurately, as it happened (but when did accuracy ever have anything to do with a good rumour!) – that all those who were traditionally 'trained' were going to have to top-up their existing qualification to a diploma level one. There was also a very real concern that even if 'the powers that be' didn't make the acquisition of an upgraded qualification a requirement, employers would go for those with the better academic qualification. It was, after all, a time of fairly poor employment prospects, with a lot of reduction of staff, disguised under a number of euphemisms such as down-sizing, rationalization, and skill-mix initiatives. No wonder that many saw the changes which were now being proposed to post-registration education, following comparatively quickly on the heels of major changes to pre-registration education, as a significant threat.

In order to combat this very real and understandable concern, the UKCC was keen to ensure that as much as possible was done to support those already in practice – either by making them feel secure and comfortable with their existing knowledge and skills, or by helping them to acquire additional qualifications, with maximum recognition of previous learning where possible, or, if feasible, a reduction in the gap that had to be crossed between existing qualifications and the new ones. In pursuit of these objectives, the UKCC agreed, on the recommendation of the education committee, for the purposes of the transitional period only (i.e. in the period between the old system of recordable qualifications being phased out and the new programmes of specialist practice being introduced, between October 1995 and October 1998) that the new programmes of education could be accepted for recording, at diploma as well as degree level. This proviso could only apply to programmes where previously no recordable qualifications existed, e.g. general practice nursing. This position was adopted to assist those for whom the opportunity to acquire a recordable qualification had not previously existed. This was a comparatively uncontentious part of the work undertaken at the time.

Where the real difficulty started was in agreeing what the position would be in relation to existing practitioners and putting into place what became known colloquially as the 'transitional arrangements'. A genuine commitment had been given throughout the whole PREPP project to the idea of offering as much recognition as possible to those individuals who had been working in professional practice, often for many years, acquiring large amounts of useful knowledge and skills, yet not necessarily having undertaken additional certificated learning or having 'anything to show' for what they had done (their words, not mine). During all of the consultation on PREPP, a very clear and understandable message had been coming through from practitioners: they did not want to have to jump through additional hoops and repeat learning – and possibly even qualifications – which they had already undertaken, merely because a new system was coming into place. There was a lot of sympathy with that view, both within the PREPP steering groups whilst the work was underway and also amongst the Council and National Board members and officers. They all wanted to acknowledge the good work done by practitioners on a daily basis and they also recognized that to expect people to do additional unnecessary and repetitive study was both insulting and expensive. The difficulty was how to give effect to that philosophy. As you would expect, the result was a compromise, and like all compromises it didn't suit everybody!

One of the difficulties was the fact that there are a lot of players in this particular game, all with different roles and responsibilities and different levels of autonomy. Detailed information on the credit accumulation scheme (CATS) and the assessment of prior (experiential) learning (AP(E)L) can be found in Chapter 7, but it is worth just reminding ourselves briefly at this stage of who does what.

The setting of standards for registrable or recordable professional qualifications in nursing, midwifery and health visiting lies with the UKCC, in its legislation or guidelines. Such standards could include, for example, a statement that maximum credit can be allowed for previous learning. In other words, that gives the legislative 'permission' for such activity. This always has to be the first step. The National Boards then issue guidance on the detail of course/programme standards which goes out to individual institutions. An institution will then submit either a course or a 'package' of courses for approval, seeking approval to run both specific courses and, potentially, others, providing they meet the overall standards set down. Approval is by means of approval visits made by National Board officers, where the detail of the curriculum, number and type of staff, clinical placements, assessments and so on are considered. The programmes are then either agreed, modified, or not approved. This can be done either for individual programmes or, more commonly now, on the basis of the approval of the institution. In relation to the award of credit, for example, the National Boards would ensure, as part of the approval mechanism, that there are processes in place for the claiming and the award of credit. This is the 'professional' element of the process, which is an integral part of the academic process.

However, as you know, all pre- and post-registration nursing, midwifery and health visiting programmes are now delivered in institutions of higher education, which, being autonomous institutions, have their own requirements and rules for academic issues such as the award of credit. For example, some institutions will say that that however much relevant previous study an individual has undertaken, a minimum of $x\%$ of the actual course must be actually taught in order to ensure integration and synthesis of knowledge. The amount of credit varies from institution to institution – it may be as high as 75% in some places, but will be much lower in others. So you can see that recognition of previous learning can be quite a complex business.

There is also the issue of the actual mechanics of how one claims credit. Some institutions – mainly those from the old polytechnic sector, although the 'traditional' institutions are catching up fast – have very sophisticated mechanisms in place for claiming and being awarded credit. In others, it can be difficult to do. How you demonstrate previous learning will also vary – in some places you have to submit an essay (or several); in other places, assessment may be on the basis of a portfolio of previous work, e.g. case studies; in yet others, an interview may suffice. Although there have been moves to streamline such activity, each institution likes to guard its own standards, so students must expect variation and inconsistency. The good news is that it does mean that if you have the opportunity to shop around you will definitely gain more credit in some places than others.

With all this in mind, a working group was set up of Council and Board officers, to make proposals regarding:

- the recognition of existing qualifications
- the position of those who did not want to undertake further study
- the acquisition of credit for those who wanted to undertake a new specialist qualification.

Any such proposals had to take into account both the letter and spirit of what had already been said during the discussion and consultation phase of PREP. This immediately ruled out what would undoubtedly have been by far the neatest and tidiest option, which was to 'draw a line in the sand' between the old and the new systems and say that the only way to get a specialist qualification was to do one of the new programmes – end of story! There were a lot of people who supported that particular view, as they thought (rightly, of course) that any compromise position would run the risk of diluting professional and academic standards. However, this was *not* an option, given the commitments that had already beeen made, so alternative routes had to be found. After a lot of hard work, the following position was agreed.

Use of the specialist practitioner title

The UKCC would not require registered nurses to undertake additional study to work as a specialist practitioner, provided that:

- they have a post-registration clinical qualification following a course of 4 months or more in length (including all school nursing qualifications) relevant to their area of practice
- they and their employer are confident that they have the skills and knowledge safely and effectively to fulfil their role as defined in the UKCC's documents *Scope of Professional Practice* and *Code of Professional Conduct.*

Under these circumstances, the UKCC is content that such individuals may use the title 'specialist practitioner', provided that the practitioner and their employer are satisfied with the arrangements. Such arrangements will not, however, result in a new qualification or any new entry on the UKCC's register. It is important to be aware that these arrangements only apply where the previous qualification(s) and experience are relevant to the role being undertaken.

A nurse may need to undertake additional studies or experience, if their qualification is not relevant to the current area of practice or if the qualification has not been consolidated by appropriate recent and relevant experience. It also means that if such an individual wishes to move from their current post, any new employer may have different criteria for employment or different expectations of the qualifications to be held by their employees.

Other recordable qualifications

During the transitional period until 31 October 1998, the UKCC would, at the request of a National Board, continue to record qualifications obtained following successful completion of an approved course. This included new qualifications that have not been previously approved for recording.

These qualifications will not meet the requirements for specialist qualifications set out above and so those receiving the qualifications will not be automatically entitled to call themselves a specialist practitioner. However, if such an individual records such a qualification during the transitional period and they meet the requirements set out above, they may be eligible to use the *title* of specialist practitioner. Such qualifications could also be used as credit towards the specialist practitioner qualification, in due course, if an individual ever decides that they wish to do more studying.

Specialist qualifications

The new specialist qualifications can only be obtained by satisfactorily completing a course approved by a National Board, to the UKCC's standards described earlier in the chapter.

The use of titles

There is no doubt that the plethora of titles in use across the health care professions is potentially confusing for individual patients and clients, employers, other health care workers and the general public. It is not, of course, an issue confined to health – we have all come across an increasing number of examples of the expanded use of title and probably all know plumbers who call themselves heating consultants and dustmen known as refuse operatives, to name but two. No doubt many readers can still remember the angst created amongst the medical profession the first time that nurses had the temerity to refer to themselves as consultants. On the subject of terminology, I still remember with amusement the response from a doctor to the Project 2000 consultation who wrote in high dudgeon about the 'new-fangled tendency to refer to patients as "clients" '. According to him, only two professions had clients – solicitors and prostitutes!

There is, however, a real issue here, which is about misleading those for whom we care – inadvertently or otherwise. One of the purposes of PREP was to try and make sense of the plethora of titles in use. As far as the UKCC was concerned, it was about linking titles to specific qualifications recorded on the UKCC register, as a benchmark of quality – so that it would be explicit and clear what experience/qualifications an individual possessed in order to use a particular title. This is an area studded with potential landmines because there is very little legal protection offered to very many titles in use, in health, let alone elsewhere. Most importantly, and in my view very regrettably, not even the word 'nurse' is protected in law. It is only the notion of 'registration' that is protected and where individuals can be prosecuted if they intend to deceive. In effect, this means that employers or individuals can use whatever title or descriptor they choose for a particular job – with the resultant potential confusion. Midwives do have greater protection with a specific definition of the title 'midwife'.

One of the groups who have suffered most from this 'flexibility' are nurse practitioners. This book is not the place for an erudite and lengthy discussion of the concept of the nurse practitioner, but the fact is that there are a lot of registered nurses who call themselves nurse practitioners and a lot of nurses employed in posts called nurse practitioner posts. The problem is – what does this mean? There is a 1 year course offered by the Royal College of Nursing called a nurse practitioner course, but not everyone who calls themselves a nurse practitioner has completed this, or indeed any other, course or specific preparation. And, conversely, not everyone who has completed the course is employed as a nurse practitioner. This was an issue debated regularly during the PREP discussions. It was not resolved in any satisfactory way – other than by its omission – in the standards agreed in March 1994, and as a result had to be returned to time and again in the ensuing years. It was a major feature of the 'listening exercise' on advanced practice undertaken by the UKCC in 1996–97.

CONCLUSION

This chapter has looked at the setting up of the PREPP project and the significant stages of its work. It has also looked in some detail at the implementation of the proposals, to help you understand how the current requirements came into place. Hopefully, it has given you some insight into the policy-making process and the complexity of the activity that has to take place when considering a change as significant as that of the PREP proposals.

REFERENCES

HMSO 1990 The NHS and Community Care Act. HMSO, London
HMSO 1995 The Nurse, Midwives and Health Visitors (Periodic Registration) Rules Amendment Order 1995 SI 967. HMSO, London
UKCC 1986 Project 2000: a new preparation for practice. UKCC, London
UKCC 1990 The report of the post registration education and practice project (discussion document). UKCC, London
UKCC 1993a Consultation on the council's standards for post registration. UKCC, London
UKCC 1993b Registrar's letter 1/1993 – the council's position concerning a period of support and preceptorship. UKCC, London
UKCC 1994 The future of professional practice – the council's standards for education and practice following registration (PREP) – position statement (number 1), March 1994. UKCC, London
UKCC 1995a The future of professional practice – the council's standards for education and practice following registration (PREP) – position statement (number 2), March 1995. UKCC, London
UKCC 1995b Registrar's letter 3/1995 – the council's position concerning a period of support and preceptorship. UKCC, London
UKCC 1997 PREP and you. UKCC, London

6

The PREP requirements

Soap and education are not as sudden as a massacre, but they are as deadly in the long run.

(*A Curious Dream*, Mark Twain)

INTRODUCTION

My guess is that this is the chapter most people will turn to first. And why not? To an extent, the rest of the book is irrelevant unless you are comfortable with the actual requirements and what they will mean to you on a day-to-day basis. After all, the most important question for most readers will be: 'Have I done all that I need to, to renew my registration?' So, let's get that clear right now.

You may well ask why this chapter is not first in the book – indeed, there would have been some arguments for having done so. However, what I hope that you will have realized by now, is that the purpose of this book is to put the actual mechanics of the PREP requirements into the broader context of lifelong learning, the increasing changes to the way society is organizing its work and the growing movement for continuing professional development. Presented in this way, I think it helps to see why and when the Council undertook the work that it did. I hope that it will also have helped those individual registrants who still think that putting specific requirements in place for registration, beyond paying a fee, is 'a cheek' and 'one more thing to have to worry about at a time when everyone is having a go at us' (a very brief selection of some of the comments I have heard on my travels) to see why staying up to date is so important.

One of the things I have always found when talking about PREP is that individuals have the greatest difficulty believing that the requirements are so flexible. This, I believe, is entirely understandable. If you have read the previous chapters, you will know that this approach has been adopted because the UKCC was trying, in its attitude to PREP, to 'regulate' the professions in as flexible, innovative, yet 'adult' way as possible. The approach was based on the fact that all the individuals on the register are professionally accountable, responsible individuals, who all practice under the principles set out in their code of professional conduct. However, to be blunt, this is not a mind-set with which everyone was, or is yet, comfortable. This is hardly surprising, given that there are over 640 000 registered nurses, midwives and health visitors on the register, the vast majority of whom were 'trained' in a period when obedience to authority, especially that of authority to one's seniors in the hierarchy – and to the medics – was paramount. Independent thought and decision-making was not high on the agenda of many 'training schools'. The general nursing councils and the central midwives boards, for example, had explicit and exact rules, which had to be obeyed. This is indeed how all the professions were 'governed', and nursing and midwifery were probably stricter than many. This is not an issue to be lightly dismissed when considering how people approach meeting their PREP requirements. It comes as quite a shock – sometimes a most uncomfortable one – to be told that there is no absolute right or wrong way of doing things. Choice and flexibility can be uncomfortable bedfellows. For a start, it can take longer! It is often much easier to be 'told' what to do – what course to attend, what personal profile to use, what cost is attached to a particular activity – than to be given the freedom to decide for oneself. The approach was not chosen to make people feel uncomfortable, however, but to treat the nurses, midwives and health visitors on the professional register like responsible professionals and to make it easier in practice to meet the requirements, without having to be tied down into a rigid, expensive, inflexible process.

So what do all those of us on the register have to do to meet the PREP requirements?

WHAT DOES 'PRACTISING' OR 'IN PRACTICE' MEAN?

This is the first question to be answered. Are you 'practising' in PREP terms in your current or proposed role? Do you actually need to be registered for the job you are doing? The answer will vary, and it lies with you the practitioner. The main thing to remember is that PREP is intended to be as *inclusive* as possible. It is hoped that as many people as possible will want to maintain their registration. It is in no-one's interest, least of all the UKCC's, that thousands of people lose their registration. 'Practise', therefore, is intended to be interpreted very broadly. It is certainly *not* intended to embrace only those engaging in clinical activity, although this is a common misinterpretation. In other words, if you are using your nursing, midwifery or health visiting qualification in some way, then the UKCC would expect you to maintain your registration. The legislation says that for a person to be treated as 'practising' he/she 'must be working *in some capacity* by virtue of their nursing, midwifery or health visiting qualification as the case may be'. (Section 22(1), The Nurses, Midwives and Health Visitors Act 1997).

This broad definition does mean, of course, that there will be those on the register who legitimately maintain their registration, within the context of PREP, but do not necessarily maintain their clinical competence. This is an important distinction to draw, to avoid misunderstanding. Such individuals would not be required to complete a statutory return to practice programme if they were re-entering clinical practice. They would, however, within the responsibilities set out in their code of conduct, have to ensure that they were competent to undertake the work in hand. Many responsible individuals – and, indeed, a responsible employer – would consider in those circumstances that the individual needs some form of informal reorientation programme, even if a formal programme is not a statutory requirement.

Let us look at some examples of who should be maintaining registration. Some, of course, are easy. If you are working as a D grade staff nurse in an acute surgical ward, then you are obviously practising; equally obviously you need your registration to be employed, and you need to meet the PREP requirements to maintain that registration. Similarly, if you are employed as one of that endangered species of nurse or midwife managers, you need to meet the requirements. If you are a practising midwife (as defined in the *Midwives Rules*, UKCC 1993a) you must meet the PREP requirements. If you hold a teaching post, teaching nursing, midwifery or community nursing, then you must meet the requirements.

So far, so good. Life, however, is rarely that simple. Increasingly, individuals are employed in roles where the position is not so clear. What about the ever growing number of nurses, who are employed by the social services, as the boundaries between social care and nursing care become ever more blurred?

The answer lies with the individual. If you are of the opinion that you use your nursing, midwifery or health visiting qualification, in some capacity, in your daily work, then you will want to maintain your registration. Let me use myself as an example. When I was working at the UKCC, it was quite clear that I needed my registration, as it was a requirement of my position as director of standards promotion that I was a registered nurse and/or midwife. The decision had already been taken for me. My next role was working as a consultant in professional standards and development, and here I had no-one else to make the decision. The answer, however, was quite clear to me. It was essential that I maintain my registration, in order to have the necessary knowledge and skills to undertake my new role with credibility and competence. Therefore, like everyone else who needs their registration, I have to meet my PREP requirements.

A few more examples. If you are the owner of a nursing home you are not required by law to be a registered nurse. If you are a matron of a nursing home, you are required to be. The position in relation to PREP is then clear. If you are a nursing home matron, you must meet PREP. If you are an owner, who happens to be a nurse – as many are – you have to decide whether your qualification is relevant in relation to your current role. You may well decide that it is not and that you will therefore choose not to maintain registration.

What about a nurse with a qualification in the care of people with a learning disability? Such individuals are increasingly being employed by social services and are well aware that a nursing qualification may not be a requirement for the role. Indeed, their predecessor or successor may well not have one. *Again, the answer must lie with the individual*. If you are of the view that you are using your nursing qualification – and I am sure many of you would be – then you will choose to maintain your registration and meet the PREP requirements.

Let us now look at a slightly more contentious area – the residential care sector. A large number of individuals with nursing qualifications are employed in this sector, although the legislation does not allow them to be employed *as* registered nurses because the home is licensed to give social, not nursing, care. Should these individuals maintain their registration? Here, the UKCC's position remains flexible and believes that the answer should lie with the individual, even though this position does not sit entirely comfortably with the legislation of the Registered Homes Act 1984. Many individuals working in this sector will consider that they are giving nursing care, even though it may be under the indirect supervision of the district nurse or general practitioner, after appropriate assessment of individual's knowledge and competence. They will then choose to maintain their registration by meeting the PREP requirements.

What about a health visitor who is working as a health education officer? Depending on the exact nature of the work and their client group, they may well decide that they are using their health visiting qualification in some capacity and will therefore have to maintain their registration with the UKCC.

Unwaged experience

One of the questions the UKCC was frequently asked, once the PREP requirements became public, was about individuals who, through no fault of their own, are not currently waged because they have given up paid work and are using their nursing qualifications in their own home, to care for a dependant. This was a question which often came in on the helpline, frequently, although not exclusively, affecting female nurses in their 40s and 50s who had every intention of returning to paid work once their circumstances changed. They did not, in the meantime, want their registration to lapse.

In June 1996, the UKCC agreed to extend the notion of being 'in practice', to include unwaged experience, providing certain criteria are met (UKCC 1996a). PREP in practice terms, therefore, now includes the delivery of nursing care in an unwaged capacity to a friend, relative or dependant provided that:

- the assessment, planning and implementation of physical or psychological care is involved
- the services of a professional carer or in-patient care would be required if the individual were not available.

The individual registrant would be required to keep a record of their experience in their personal professional profile. They would also be required to complete the necessary PREP study activity and should choose something which is relevant to their registration and role. Providing that these requirements are met, an individual would not be required to undertake a statutory return to practice programme, even if their period(s) of unwaged experience exceeded 5 years.

To answer the question frequently asked, albeit, equally frequently, tongue-in-cheek: 'No, staying at home to bring up your children does not constitute unwaged experience within the PREP definition.' It just feels like it!

This expansion of existing policy is a good example of how the UKCC has been responsive to registrants whilst creating its flexible but meaningful standards policies.

So, having considered the concept of 'practice' in some detail, let us turn to the actual requirements themselves.

SUMMARY OF PREP REQUIREMENTS

It may come as a surprise to some readers to be reminded that there are, in fact, four major sets of requirements relating to the UKCC's standards for education and practice following registration. These are:

- standards for a period of support for newly registered practitioners, under the guidance of a preceptor
- standards for maintaining registration
- standards for return to practice programmes
- standards for specialist practice.

Although all of these standards will be of interest to the reader, it is only the second set which is relevant to *every* individual on the register and has the force of legislation behind it. Let us look at the standards for preceptorship first, followed by those for maintaining registration and then those for return to practice programmes.

Specialist practice will be dealt with in the next chapter.

Standards for a period of support for newly registered practitioners under the guidance of a preceptor

All practitioners are accountable for their practice from the moment of registration. However, throughout the whole period of discussion and debate during the PREP project, the issue of support for newly qualified practitioners kept reoccurring, time and again. Not only was it an issue for the Council members and the project steering group but also for all those with whom we were in contact. There was a very real, frequently repeated, message, that those who were newly qualified needed the support of a more experienced colleague for those early, rather uncertain months of professional practice.

It was certainly not, as has subsequently been suggested by a few cynical commentators, a 'crutch' put into place to support inadequately prepared 'Project 2000' registrants. If necessary, this argument can be comprehensively dismissed by a look at the timing. The PREP project got underway at the beginning of 1990 and reported in 1994. The requirements for a period of preceptorship received such widespread and unequivocal support that they were published in advance of the other PREP proposals in January 1993 (UKCC 1993b). Indeed, they had been re-evaluated and revised by January 1995 (UKCC 1995a). Project 2000 programmes only started to be run in England in the academic year of 1989 and there were no registrants through, even in the initial small numbers, until July 1992. Wales and Northern Ireland began their programmes in 1990, with the first diplomates exiting in 1993, and Scotland began in 1992, with their first diplomates exiting in 1995. So, there were no Project 2000 registrants practising until the end of 1993, and even then it was in very small numbers. PREP's final proposals were agreed in March 1994 and it was during the previous 3 years that existing practitioners had been asking for support for newly qualified registrants. In other words, for the products of the previous courses. Many people will agree that this was an issue that had needed addressing for a long time.

Interestingly, the non-nurses on the UKCC at the time were amazed that any formal steps had to be taken to support the newly qualified. I can still remember one colleague, an accountant, saying with a gently puzzled air: 'Well, surely *all* professions take steps to properly support their newly qualified?' Regrettably not, as a lot of readers can testify.

The preceptorship standards

Purpose

Being newly qualified is a transition period which can be stressful as well as exciting, as new demands are made on individuals who have until recently been students. Although professionally competent and accountable, newly registered practitioners are likely to be in need of support from their more experienced colleagues. Such support is in order to 'ensure responsibilities are not placed too soon upon a newly registered practitioner' (UKCC 1995a).

It is UKCC policy that all newly registered nurses, midwives and health visitors should be provided with a period of support, where possible under the guidance of a preceptor, for approximately the first 4 months of registered practice. It is important to be clear that such a period of support is not to be considered as an extension of the formal programmes leading to registration, as individuals will have achieved the necessary specific competencies or learning outcomes for safe and effective practice as part of the UKCC's requirements for registration.

In all its documentation the UKCC is at pains to point out that nurses, midwives and health visitors are accountable for their practice from the point of registration regardless of any support system. What should be aimed for is a balance between the individual level of responsibility and the experience of the individual. Support should be available to:

- all newly registered nurses, midwives and health visitors entering practice for the first time
- those entering a different field of practice by means of a second registrable qualification, and those returning to practice after a break of 5 years or more.

Moreover, it should apply to those working in the NHS or in the private or independent sector.

This includes those working, as increasing numbers are, as bank and agency staff. Where individuals, for whatever reason, do not move into paid employment immediately upon qualifying, the period of preceptorship will need to be delayed until such time as they do start work.

Length of support

The average length of a period of support should be 4 months. This should be subject to local agreement and will depend on the previous experience, qualifications and personal and professional abilities of the individual concerned. The length of time should be agreed between the individual and their preceptor. Since the original proposals relating to preceptorship were outlined, a lot of progress has been made on the concept of clinical supervision, and in many places preceptorship will be part and parcel of the arrangements for a longer-term process of clinical supervision, where they are in place.

Role of preceptors

Preceptors should be first level nurses or midwives who have normally had at least 12 months of experience in the same, or similar, clinical areas as the person they are supporting. Whether they work full- or part-time is irrelevant – what is important is that this is something they want to do and that they are enthusiastic about offering support to the newly qualified. The person with whom they are working will look to them as a valuable source of help, both professionally and personally, during their early months of professional practice. It is therefore important that the exact nature of the relationship is worked out to suit the two individuals concerned. This will take into account the type of unit where care is being given, the nature of the work and the experience and confidence of those involved. Both individuals will need to recognize that whatever preceptorship arrangements are in place, each practitioner is accountable for his/her own practice.

Preceptors can be chosen either from the area where the newly qualified individual is working or, in some instances, from another associated area of practice. Similarly, although usually less desirably, a preceptor may be from another profession.

Being a preceptor is something that does need specific preparation, although many people will have the aptitude and many experienced practitioners will have acquired some, if not all, of the necessary skills over time. Outcomes of any preparation must ensure that the preceptor will:

- have sufficient knowledge of the practitioner's programme leading to registration to identify current learning needs
- help the practitioner to apply knowledge to practice
- understand how practitioners integrate into a new practice setting and assist with this process
- understand and assist with the problems in the transition from pre-registration student to registered and accountable practitioner
- act as a resource to facilitate professional development.

Preceptorship standards should also be considered in the context of the discussion on the teaching of nursing, midwifery and health visiting in Chapter 5.

Standards for maintaining registration

This is the section in the book that will attract the greatest attention, I have no doubt. After all, this is the nub of PREP for the majority of practitioners. Ask anyone on the register what they know about PREP and the majority will mention 'study days' and 'profiles'. They may mention a few other things as well! So, what are the requirements?

First, a word about timing. The statutory requirements for the implementation of PREP came into force on 1 April 1995. In other words, that is when the legislation started. Should you want to refer to primary sources, the Statutory Instrument, or Rule, is The Nurses, Midwives and Health Visitors (Periodic Registration) Amendment Rules Approval Order 1995 Statutory Instrument (SI) No 976 (HMSO 1995). It is important to remember that this legislation was the go-ahead for the process to *start*. It is not the date when everyone had to start meeting the new requirements. Remember that registration cycle with the UKCC is on a 3-yearly basis. So, the PREP process started on April Fool's day 1995!

This means, in practice, that the *first* time that a nurse or health visitor renewed their registration after that date, they only had to complete the notification of practice form that the UKCC sent them and pay the registration fee. Midwives still had (and have), in addition, to complete their annual notification of intention to practice form. It is at the end of that first

3 year period, i.e. at the time of the *second* renewal, that the requirements relating to the completion of 5 days of study activity and use of a personal professional profile have to be met, for everyone on the register. The specific situation with regard to midwives, who already had legislation in place in relation to refresher courses, is set out later in this chapter.

A few examples. If your registration as a nurse expired on 1 June 1995, you would have completed a notification of practice form, which was enclosed with the registration papers sent out by the UKCC 6 weeks before your registration was due, and paid your fee. That was all you needed to do to be re-registered. By the time you were due for renewal, i.e. 3 years from that date on 1 June 1998, you would have to have completed 5 days of study activity and be using a personal professional profile. However, if your registration fell due for renewal for the first time after 1 April 1995 in March 1998, then you would not need to meet the requirements relating to study activity and using a personal professional profile until March 2001 – making you one of the last people to 'come in' to the PREP system. Many people started to meet the requirements before they were required to do so. That's good and means that you will be well up to speed by the time you are doing it 'for real'. By the time you are reading this book, everyone will be somewhere within their own personal PREP cycle. Once in, then the requirements will continue for every 3 year period of registration, until such time as you decide, for whatever reason, you don't need your registration any longer.

The requirements

The requirements are very simple. Indeed, as I have said before, I believe that one of the reasons people have some difficulty with PREP is because they can't believe that things are really as straightforward as they appear. Things don't have to be difficult and unpleasant in order to be valuable.

Every 3 years, each individual nurse, midwife or health visitor who wishes to maintain registration must:

- fill in a notification of practice form
- complete 5 days of study activity
- maintain a personal professional profile

In addition, those individuals who have been out of practice for 5 years or more must, from 1 April 2000, complete a statutory return to practice programme before returning to practice.

Let us look at each of those requirements in turn.

Notification of practice (NoP) form

This is a form provided by the UKCC. It will arrive the same time as the request for your registration fee and *must be completed*. If you do not fill it in, it means that your registration will lapse and cannot be renewed until the form, as part of the legal requirements for registration, has been completed. As your registration is, in effect, your licence to practice and you cannot work as a nurse, midwife and health visitor unless you are registered (see Being Registered, p. 134), it is vital that you do not let it lapse unnecessarily. *The UKCC will not remind you again if you do not fill your form in – it is your responsibility to do so.* You will need to complete a form:

- every 3 years when you renew registration
- if you change area of practice to one where you are using a different registrable qualification
- if you return to practice after a break.

The form is already personalized when you receive it and will have details of your name, address and registrable qualifications on one side. On the other side, you will be asked to complete a multiple-tick form, filling in what best describes your qualifications and type of practice. For example, are you practising with your nursing or your midwifery or your health visiting qualifications – or all three if you are a triple duty practitioner in Scotland? There is then a section relating to your area of practice – not north-west Reading, as someone put on an early form, but whether you are working, for example, in health visiting, long-stay mental health or a registered nursing home. This part of the form causes some problems. If every area of practice were to be listed for such professions as diverse as nursing, midwifery and health visiting there would be no end to the form itself. However, the categories are regularly reviewed over time and will be subject to change as practice itself changes.

The information received on these forms is scanned when it is received at the UKCC and the information is entered against the practitioner's name on the register. This is not just to give the UKCC staff something to do! Gradually – and for the first time – an accurate picture of the nursing and health visiting workforce is being compiled, which matches qualifications against type of work. Until this data was gathered by means of the notification of practice form, the information held on the UKCC data base in relation to nurses and health visitors was very limited – it could tell you which individual had which qualification, but not who was using those qualifications, or in what field of work. Lack of accurate information in these areas has made any systematic attempts to try and identify where shortfalls may arise in a particular field of practice, e.g. children's nursing, very difficult. Indeed, human resource planning has been based on little more than educated guesswork at times. The position, of course, was different for midwives, as much of this information was available from the annual notification of intention to practice forms.

From 1 April 1998, which is when the first practitioners were required to have met the PREP requirements, the form also includes a declaration to be signed by each registrant to the following effect:

I declare that I have completed the equivalent of five days of study activity since my last renewal of registration and maintained a personal professional profile.

The explanatory note reminds registrants that this is a formal declaration whereby the individual confirms their statutory obligations, in relation to the PREP requirements. It is the means whereby the individual, as an accountable practitioner, confirms that they have met their legal requirements for registration. It is an important declaration, not to be taken lightly.

Notification of intention to practise for midwives. In addition to the NoP form described above, all practising midwives will continue to complete a notification of intention to practise form annually. This is one of the legal requirements associated with the supervision of midwives and it remains separate from the PREP legislation.

Five days of study activity

The good news about the study activity is that you may well already be doing this, and indeed may have been doing so for some time. What does it actually entail?

Please make sure that you read the words carefully: 5 days of study or study activity, not 5 'study days'. The word *activity* is there deliberately to make sure that individuals realize that they do not have to do formal study days. Of course, you can if you want to. That may be your favourite way of learning and you may be lucky enough to work for a trust or nursing home where they put on regular study days and they all coincide exactly with your own personal learning needs. Lucky you – make the most of it! However, for the rest of us, a little more work will probably need to go into deciding how we want to meet our PREP requirements.

First the good news. Five days in 3 years is not a lot. As I said earlier, I expect that a lot of you are already doing more than that. The days can be whole or a part-time equivalent. This could mean for example, 10 'half' days, or it could mean attending a series of evening lectures that you collect up to 'make' one study day. No specific number of hours has been attached to a study day – that is deliberate, to allow a reasonable flexibility. More good news – the study does not have to be 'approved' by anyone. This is a common misunderstanding and, regrettably, has led to some people being exploited. This is usually by those who want to frighten their hearers about 'losing their registration', if they don't complete expensive study activity offered by particular commercial organizations. Don't misunderstand me, there are some excellent things on offer – really high-quality distance learning using a variety of media, some well planned and delivered study days and many innovative ideas. But, the *choice* is yours, the individual registrant. Only you can decide what is relevant for your needs.

I well remember, in the early PREP days, being asked to speak at a conference being put on by a commercial organization who clearly thought that they were about to make a 'killing' in the health field (no pun intended!).

They had planned a fair day – certainly nothing spectacular – for which they were charging delegates £250 each. And they were not even offering a speaker's fee! I certainly demanded one that day, although, as a rule, when at the UKCC, most of my PREP sessions were offered for free. I am pleased to report that not many delegates turned up and they soon stopped thinking they had found a gold mine. Come to think of it, I haven't seen them advertising for a while either.

So, if you don't have to do study days, what else might you want to do? You may decide that a planned visit to an appropriate library would be useful, in order to undertake, perhaps, a literature search on a topic of interest to you. That would be quite acceptable, providing you are clear about the objectives you have for the day and record them and the outcomes of your work in your personal professional profile. What some people are doing – and I think may be more fun, especially if, like me, you aren't very motivated if you have to do things on your own – is to get together with colleagues to discuss issues of professional relevance at that particular time. This could be in the form of a discussion on some new aspect of clinical practice, or perhaps looking at a difficult interpersonal issue that has arisen at work, or proposed changes to the way a particular aspect of care is delivered – the options are endless.

I hope that you have got the key message by now. PREP study activity does not have to be expensive or time-consuming – and, who knows, you may even enjoy it! My prediction is that a lot of people will choose to do things which have been arranged locally and 'officially', where these are available, at least for the first 3 years. After all, it's more convenient and you may feel, understandably, that they are more 'legitimate' because they have been arranged by others. Then, gradually, as everyone becomes more confident and realizes that the UKCC is not going to be coming down on them like a ton of bricks because 'they haven't done things right', everyone will get a lot more relaxed and innovative about it and we will start to see some really exciting things happening. Some are already happening. At a theatre nurses conference I spoke at early in 1995, a staff nurse from a recovery ward had already got a series of visits planned to other units, to see the new techniques they were implementing – and she was going to use these visits as her PREP activity. And this was well in advance of it being a statutory requirement for that particular individual. An excellent idea.

Study categories

The UKCC has identified five categories of study to help give people a 'shape' to choosing their activity.

Just because there are five categories, it does not mean that your 5 days have to be chosen one from each category. You can do all 5 days in one category if you prefer. The categories and examples of relevant issues are set out below:

- Patient, client and colleagues support
  —counselling techniques
  —leadership in professional practice
  —supervision of clinical practice
- Care enhancement
  —new techniques and approaches to care
  —standard setting
  —empowering clients and consumers of the service
- Practice development
  —visits to other units or places of interest relevant your role and practice
  —personal research/study
  —examining aspects of service provision
- Reducing risk
  —identifying health problems
  —health promotion
  —screening
- Education development
  —exchange arrangements
  —personal research/study
  —teaching and learning skills.

When you are planning your personal development in the form of study activity, it is helpful to do it in a systematic way. Chapter 8 looks at these issues in a lot more detail, but it is worth preempting the discussion a little here. The original PREP fact sheet, number 3, sets out some useful steps, which I repeat here, just in case you can't lay your hands on it right at this minute (what was it the dog was seen carrying to the bottom of the garden last week...?).

Firstly the fact sheet tells you 'to review your competence'. With hindsight, I think that sounds a bit pompous. What it really means is, have a good think about the things you are good at, the things that you are not so good at, and the areas where you know you really do need to add to your existing knowledge. Why not do this bit with someone else? Unless you are capable of being really objective, most of us need a bit of help identifying both our strengths and weaknesses. It certainly doesn't have to be a big, heavy session. Do it over a beer in the pub, if that's where you will both feel most comfortable. It doesn't necessarily have to be a professional colleague – it could be a friend or partner – but do make sure that the relationship can survive any possible fallout from such an exercise. PREP can be blamed for many things, but broken relationships should not be one of them.

Once this stage is over, then you can set your learning objectives more detail. Again, don't be put off by all the jargon. All it means is make a list of

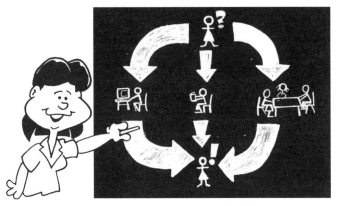

'Now you need an action plan!'

what you want to come out of any study activity. Be simple, but be realistic. You may want to get a PhD, become a really nice person, or become chief executive of the trust – but if you've only been qualified 6 months you may have some preliminary stages to go through before they become the sort of goals that you will want to commit to paper. How about 'learn more about the psychological effects of suffering from rheumatoid arthritis', or 'achieve a working knowledge of computer-held records', or 'identify three ethical issues associated with managing a surrogate pregnancy'? See – it's really quite easy (but remember, my job here is only to give you the questions, not the answers – in other words, I'm doing the easy bit).

Now you need an action plan. All this means is deciding which is the best way to achieve what you want to do. There are several things to take into account, which include, for example:

- What are your own preferences – do you work best alone or with others
- Do you have any money from any source which could help? (more on that later)
- What is already available locally?
- Are you sure that you know – have you actually asked anyone, or just sat back and said 'well, no-one told me'?
- What is the best time for you to do something – in the evening after everyone has gone to bed (if so, unless you can find other like-minded souls, it looks like distance learning for you), or perhaps it's easier at the weekend when you can arrange baby sitters, if necessary?

The hardest thing here is actually really having to think about it. By and large, nurses, midwives and health visitors are 'doers' by preference, rather than thinkers (yes, all right I know that that is a generalization, but that doesn't stop it being true!). The good news is that you do know the answers – at least you are not being asked impossible questions. You may well not have thought about it before. Even if you have undertaken this sort of analysis in the past, it might be worth trying it again because we do change our preferences over time and taking into account our different circumstances.

If you can bear some personal examples, this might show you what I mean. I know that it relates to formal study, which is well beyond what most people will want to do for PREP, but the principles are just the same. The first major studying that I undertook after my registration was the Diploma in Nursing. I did that on day release, on a part-time basis, driving to a college about 40 miles away, with the support of a helpful husband and friends who looked after the children at the end of the day. I enjoyed that very much – I had the stimulation of a taught course, yet could do the course work at home, at a time which fitted in around the family. My Diploma in Education was done on a full-time basis and required some very sophisticated child/home care arrangements, but as I had the benefit of support from family and friends it was manageable, as it only lasted for a year. I did my first degree with the Open University, however, because, at that time it was by far the most convenient way of studying because I did not have to commit myself to too much out-of-house activity at specific times, which would have been difficult to manage. I was also in a job which required a lot of train travel, so I had plenty of opportunity to read on the train. All very convenient. However, it is an experience that I would not choose to repeat, as I much prefer studying with other people regularly, rather than mainly on my own. For this reason, I chose to do a taught Master's degree. I also, unashamedly looked for one which was close to where I was working at the time, which had evening lectures, and most importantly, required minimal assessment and where I could use my current work experiences and knowledge to inform my study, thus cutting down on any duplication of work. In other words, what I had to read for 'work' informed my studies and vice versa. I think one should be quite up-front and honest about this sort of planning, otherwise things are likely to go wrong. I hope these examples from my own experience have been helpful. And just in case you thought I wasn't doing anything else at the same time as my studying, I was fitting it all in around a husband, two children, a horse, numerous dogs and cats, a full-time job, a house and a full social life!

This discussion started because we were thinking about action planning. I hope that I have got the message across that action plans, even the simplest ones, stand a much greater chance of success, if they are given a reasonable amount of thought in advance. That is not meant to sound patronising or pretentious, but realistic: when you are busy – as we all are – it is very easy to rush into things without thinking them through. A little thought is a good investment here and will save a lot of time in the end.

Having given things some thought and decided what you would ideally like to do, in order to achieve your objectives, you need to think next about who, if anyone, can help you to achieve your goals. In most instances, this is likely to be your employer. The plan with the greatest chance of success is going to be the one where your needs coincide with the needs of your workplace, and therefore, one hopes, your employer. If this is the case, it would be reasonable to expect maximum support, in terms of time off and financial assistance. You will have to be realistic. If there are two conferences on your specialist subject and one is in New York and the other is in the local postgraduate centre, you don't need me to tell you which one you are likely to be going to! On the other hand, if there is not a lot available in your area of speciality and it is an essential part of the organization's business, then who knows where you may end up.

Once you have chosen an activity and completed it, what happens next? This is where PREP differs from virtually all other continuing education systems. The UKCC could have a chosen a system whereby all one had to do was to record one's presence at an event – the 'smartie/brownie points' approach. This is all that a lot of other systems require. However, we all know that there is no correlation whatsoever between the number of hours that we sit in front of a lecturer, or reading an erudite tome, and the amount of learning received. Who was it who said that the knowledge lecturers impart goes from the mouth of the lecturer, down the students' arms to their pens, to their paper, without once engaging the brain of either party? We have all been in that class, haven't we, as student or speaker, at some stage in our lives? So, what is different about PREP?

Remember what PREP set out to do. It was to put a framework in place which enables practitioners to maintain and develop their professional knowledge and competence. So, the study that you choose has to be relevant to your registration and your role. In other words, it's about you choosing things that help you to do your job even better. If you are not currently working, then choose something relevant to your last area of work, or where you hope to work next. So, once you've chosen and completed the study activity, you need to record it in your personal professional profile. This is what the profile is about – making the link between the activity that you undertake and the effect that it has on your professional practice. I think that this bit is actually quite difficult, at least to get started, and there is certainly no specific right or wrong way to do it – no 'approved UKCC' method of profile completion! There is, however, some useful advice in the original fact sheets (UKCC 1994a) and in the booklet produced by the UKCC in the autumn of 1997 called *PREP and You* (UKCC 1997a).

Personal professional profile (PPP)

I think that the completion of the PPP is the thing that most people worry about. In a survey carried out by the *Nursing Times* and Queen's Nursing Institute (Dilloway et al 1997), one respondent wrote: 'I have no idea how to complete my personal profile and would find information on this most helpful'. Having sympathized, I would suggest that anyone in a similar position will find the information produced by the UKCC, either in the original fact sheets or in the booklet entitled *PREP and You* (UKCC 1997a). Let us have a look at it in more detail here.

The main function of a personal professional profile is as a record of your career progress and professional development. It will contribute to your professional development by helping you to 'recognize, understand and value your abilities, strengths, achievements and experiences'. It also acts as an easily available source of information, to be used at any time. How often have you wished that you had all the facts about the dates of your various periods of employment, qualifications and so on, all together in one place. For those of you with your CVs all beautifully up-to-date, on disk and in hard copy in your PPP, please go off and make a cup of coffee at this stage: you don't need to read the rest of this section – and well done, by the way! My guess is, however, that there will be a few people who are still with me. If it's any consolation, let me tell you about my profile. Yes, I do have one – so that's stage one successfully achieved. Which one? One that I was given on my PREP travels that I happened to like best, in terms of layout and colour and the fact that it has a tree on it. You see, decisions about which profile to use do not have to be based on well documented and researched data – I just happened to like the tree! There is no official UKCC profile. The Council was often asked why it did not produce its own profile. It certainly was the original intention to have one available from the UKCC. The decision was made mainly to allow people maximum flexibility, in terms of what they could choose. Some like to have large, impressive looking documents, with loads of inserts which virtually tell them what to think and write on every line; others are quite content to have a colourful 'cheapie' from the local newsagents, that they can then customize. Still others – and I guess, in increasing numbers – will want to store the information electronically. In fact, that's probably what I will do in the end, now that I have all the enthusiasm of the new convert for my new, all-singing, all-dancing PC. I'll keep the 'tree' one as a repository for all the paperwork, until I have time to get it all on floppy disk. The format doesn't matter, it's the concept that's important.

So, what needs to go into the file? I was touched by the quote, also from the survey that I've just mentioned, from the practitioner who rather plaintively said: 'I feel that after 20 years of nursing and midwifery, my past counts for nothing. I am also unable to remember what I have done or achieved.' I have good news for him/her in several respects. Certainly the individual's past counts for something. It is what has made them the competent, experienced, knowledgeable practitioner that they are now. There is nothing in PREP that will, or indeed should, diminish that. The second piece of good news is even better. I doubt if many of us could remember all the things we have done in the last 20 years. Fortunately, there is no reason why you should need to do so. The personal professional profile associated with PREP is about each 3 year registration period and the study activity you have

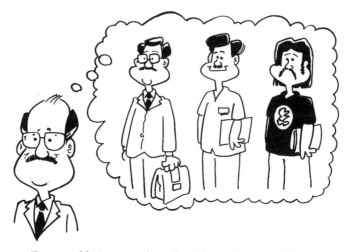

'I am unable to remember what I have done or achieved!'

undertaken in each 3 year period. So, once you have got all the basic data together, you only have to keep a comparatively brief record. Let us look at that in more detail.

What is a profile? People write dissertations on the semantic differences between 'profiles' and 'portfolios'. You will be relieved to hear that I am not going to do so. Basically, your profile is a flexible, comprehensive account of your personal development and how that has been achieved. It is more than a curriculum vitae, although much of what you would find in a CV will be in your profile, for convenience if for no other reason. Your CV will contain details of your formal education, professional qualifications and work experience. A portfolio is usually what is compiled when you are seeking credit towards a particular qualification or award. It would therefore hold information on things like educational and professional achievements and records of anything you have written or published, such as articles or papers. A lot of this information will also be held in your profile – it is much easier to have it all together, after all.

But the PPP envisaged by the UKCC is more than that. Remember what I said earlier about PREP being more than the collection of x number of hours of study, about how it is trying to move that one step further (albeit a huge step) to looking at how that study actually helps you to maintain and develop your professional knowledge and competence. So the profile goes beyond mere descriptions of achievements. It will be about actively reflecting on and recording what you learn from your activities – what may happen both on a day-to-day basis and as a result of your planned activities. The most important thing, however, is that it is a personal document about *you*. A large amount of the information in it will be private and confidential to you. It is for you to choose whether you share the information directly with anyone.

Some people will be quite happy to share its contents, others would rather not – that is your choice. There will be some parts that will have to be available for the UKCC for audit purposes in due course, but these will be the descriptive parts, indicating what study activity has been undertaken, as well as the lessons learned.

However you decide to organize your profile, there is certain basic information that it needs to contain. My suggestion would be, that if you are starting to compile your own profile for the first time, this is where you should start. It's often easier to start with gathering factual information.

Record of factual information

- Personal information (biographical details)
- Registrable qualifications, such as registered nurse, registered midwife
- Recordable qualifications, such as specialist practitioner (medical nursing)
- Other academic or professional qualifications, such as degrees or diplomas
- Positions held throughout your career, in chronological order, starting with your current post
- Other interests, activities and positions that you have held, in addition to your paid job.

This is all information that you will already have available somewhere, even if only in your memory, although it may take a bit of time to drag it out accurately. You will probably have to play around with times and dates for a while, until they make sense. Unless you have been a meticulous keeper of such records over the years – and most of us aren't – it is amazingly easy to forget large chunks of time or to get the dates in a muddle.

Self-appraisal of professional performance. This part is not as easy. As I said earlier on in this chapter, this activity may best be done together with someone else. However you do it, you need to consider and record:

- the things that you are good at
- the areas where you want/need to enhance your knowledge/skills
- your personal and professional achievements
- notes from your analysis of significant events

Record of goals and action plans. As we discussed earlier, this is an area where you will need to have thought through, in advance, what you want to do. Be realistic, don't set targets that you know you can't meet – that will only make you feel like a failure if you don't achieve them. But don't make them too easy either; you need to stretch yourself, so that you get a sense of achievement when you have finished. Make sure that you record, at least, the following:

- Your goals, action plans, a time-scale for achieving them and a schedule of dates when you will review progress.

- Each time you review your goals, describe and record your progress. If necessary, revise your action plan.
- Record the outcomes of your action plans as you achieve them.

Record of formal learning. This is a fairly straightforward bit and is the part that many people are already doing. Again, it may take a while to gather the information for the first time, but once you get into the habit, then it will become second nature (eventually!). Make sure that you document all your formal learning activities, including details of:

- study days/seminars, courses and conferences that you attend
- visits to other places of interest or units, which are relevant to your work
- time spent in the library, e.g. carrying out a literature search on a topic of interest which is of interest to you and which is relevant to your work.

And this is the key issue – in relation to each of these events described above, then you need to describe and record, for each one:

- its relevance to your professional practice and development
- what you hope to achieve from it
- your assessment of the outcomes of the activities
- the time spent on each activity, together with any follow-up work.

Reflective practice. There are lots of books on the market on reflective practice. It has become very much the fashion, particularly for the practice-based professions. If you think you don't know anything about it, don't worry. To an extent it is like many things – giving a smart title to something that you may already know how to do, but have never given it a name. It is an important concept however, and needs to be thought about a little further. 'The relationship between the way that nurses think and the actions they perform is one of the key debates in the nursing profession' (Lauder 1994; see also Cervero 1988). The chief proponent of reflective practice is Donald Schon (1983, 1987). He argues that the competent professional cannot simply apply textbook principles and solutions to a given problem, but that innovative and creative actions need to be designed for each unique problem. In this way a link is made between 'thinking' and 'doing'. Others, for example Kolb (1984), would argue that practice and theory are separated, in that all learning begins with experience which students must then reflect on, and on the basis of that thinking gain new insights, information, understanding and ways of solving problems. Many of you will have sympathy with Lauder (1994) who considers that what appears to be missing from the reflective concept is 'the bridge between thinking about care and actually caring.'

What does all this mean to you in practice and in relation to completing your own personal professional profile? Not a lot, you may think. But it is relevant. Never mind whose theory you support, there is a useful process hidden in here. The ability to appraise your own performance and the standards of your own professional knowledge and competence is essential. Using the technique of critical reflection, or critical incident analysis, is useful here, thinking about a particular event. Choose an event that was particularly significant for you, either because it was particularly successful or because it may have been particularly difficult and may not have been resolved very satisfactorily. Then you need to methodically review the event. First of all, describe what happened. Note any challenges which emerged. Who dealt with them and how? What was your role – were you the one who provided the solution, the one who got people talking, the one who took the necessary action, or, on this occasion, were you the one who had to stand back and let others solve the problem? Then go on to identify what you learnt from the situation and reflect on how, and in what way, the experience has affected your professional practice. It may be that as a result of this type of activity you identify some new goals for the future – some new knowledge that you may wish to acquire, for example, in terms of people management. Remember, PREP defines practice as a very broad concept. So what is described here can be applied to whatever job you are doing with your nursing, midwifery or health visiting qualification.

As I said earlier, you may find that this is easier to do with someone else, at least until you become really skilled at doing it – even then, you may find that it is more fun with others.

Profiles in Welsh

Even in advance of the requirements of the Welsh Language Act 1993 (HMSO 1993), which requires that 'parity of esteem' is given to the Welsh and English languages, the UKCC had discussed the issue of completing personal professional profiles in Welsh. It was agreed that this would, of course, be acceptable and when any Welsh profiles are brought in the audit process, then the Council will bear the costs of translation. This facility is not available in any other language.

Access to profile information

This matter is important enough to return to again, briefly. As was said earlier, your profile is your own personal property. The information within it is private to you, although there will be elements of it that you have to share with the UKCC, in order to demonstrate, on request, that you have met the minimum statutory requirements in relation to the completion of 5 days of study. This information only ever needs to go to the UKCC when they request it, by the way. Many rumours abound about UKCC officers descending on unsuspecting practitioners demanding to see their profiles. Don't believe a word of it – these are just nasty rumours put out by those who like to frighten children with stories of strange creatures under the bed! Rumour is always more fun than the truth! Once the arrangements are in place for audit of profiles – and remember this can't be until 2001, when everyone is brought into PREP – then you may receive a request for details of elements of your profile. But again, don't worry – there will have been plenty of advanced warning from the UKCC on what will be expected.

Lots of questions have been asked about whether the contents of a profile could be subpoenaed for legal purposes. In theory, yes, they could, but their usefulness would be so limited that they would be virtually valueless. After all, there will no means of identifying individual patients as any information of that nature would have been presented without names anyway. The other question frequently asked is whether employers have right of access to your profile. The answer is an unequivocal 'no, they do not' – it is your own personal property. Having said that, of course, there are some provisos – there always are, aren't there? Some Trusts are providing profiles to their staff and are intending to use them as part of the local individual performance review process. That is not what the PREP profiles are about, so you have a decision to make. You may decide that you are comfortable with these arrangements – and you may be. It depends on the way that IPR is used where you work. If it is implemented in a supportive, positive way then there will be no problem. If this is the case, you may then decide to use your 'work' profile as your personal professional profile for PREP purposes. Things may not be as comfortable as that, however, and you may have to decide that the only answer is to have two separate documents, if your employer is going to require completion of a profile as part of your terms and conditions of service and you are not happy about putting some of your 'PREP' things in it. Of course, this is not an ideal solution because there would be some duplication but it need not be a major problem – it's easy enough to copy things, if necessary.

Audit of profile information

Understandably, this is an issue which really worries registrants. Please be reassured. The responsibility lies with the UKCC to guide you through the type and presentation of material that it may ask you to submit, at such time as you are brought into the audit process. A variety of audit tools will be piloted by the UKCC from 1998 to 2000. This will help to inform the method which is finally chosen for formal use from 1 April 2001 onwards. The data received from both the pilots and the real audits will help to provide a basis for the standards for both pre- and post-registration education in the future, and provide an opportunity for registrants to explore the relevance of their learning.

Return to practice programmes

It is interesting, but I think not surprising, that this element of the PREP proposals was agreed long before any other part. I suppose that, in terms of staying up-to-date, which after all is what PREP is really about, it is easy for everyone to agree, in principle, that if you have actually not been using your qualification(s) for several years then you are likely to need some sort of refresher 'course', to ensure that you are, at the very least, safe before you start practising again, in whatever capacity. This is one of the 'common sense' decisions that found a lot of favour amongst all those involved in the discussions. The discussion, of course, related specifically to nurses and health visitors, as midwives had had the advantage of statutory refresher courses for many years (see below for further details). It was helpful to have their knowledge and experience to draw on, when thinking about widening the requirements to all those on the professional register. Interestingly, there had previously been no statutory requirements for health visitor refresher courses, although custom and practice had evolved a system of 5-yearly 'refreshers' which many health visitors attended as good practice. Indeed, many did think they were a legislative requirement. They were, in fact, mandatory.

To an extent, the decision to use a 5 year 'break' was an arbitrary one, although it seemed sensible to use the same period of time as midwives had already established. A number of people have asked why a 3 year period was not chosen, to mirror the registration period, but given that the two periods were unlikely to coincide (i.e. someone conveniently having their 3 year break in practice to neatly coincide with their 3 year period of registration), there seemed to be little advantage. Also 3 years is a very short period in an individual's professional life span.

So, what was finally decided?

The purpose of return to practice programmes

Return to practice programmes are designed to ensure that practitioners seeking to renew their registration 're-enter practice with up-to-date competence, current skills and confidence in order to maintain safe and effective standards of patient and client care' (UKCC 1995b, 1996b).

Start date for statutory programmes

From 1 April 2000, all practitioners returning to practice after a break (see below) have to complete a return to practice programme before they can return, using their nursing, midwifery and health visiting qualification.

Break in practice

A break in practice for nurses and health visitors is defined as practising with a particular registered qualification for fewer than 100 working days, or 750 hours, in a 5 year period. This same definition applies to midwives from 1 April 2000 (see below). One hundred working days can also be interpreted as 100 working 'sessions' to accommodate those practitioners, such as family planning nurses, who practise for shorter periods, but nonetheless regularly. The 100 working days do not have to total 750 hours – they are offered as alternatives, to accommodate different ways of working and to ensure maximum flexibility.

The position for midwives

Rule 37 of the UKCC *Midwives Rules* (November 1993) had for many years required all midwives wishing to return to practice and who had not practised as a midwife for at least the equivalent of 12 working weeks during the preceding 5 years to attend a National Board approved course of practical and theoretical instruction of at least 4 weeks. The Rule 37 requirements apply to midwives until 1 April 2000. The reason for the difference between this requirement and the new ones for nurses and health visitors is the definition of a break in practice. The Rule 37 definition related to 12 working weeks, whereas the new definition relates to 100 working days, which is 20 working weeks. A 5 year phase-in period was therefore planned to ensure that no midwives were disadvantaged by the introduction of the new rule.

Midwives refresher courses and PREP

Transitional arrangements were introduced by the UKCC to make sure that midwives would not have to undertake the PREP requirements of 5 days of study activity *in addition* to the refresher requirements set out in Rule 37 of the *Midwives Rules*. The transitional arrangements only apply to those midwives who would otherwise have to meet the PREP requirements as well as the refresher course requirements. The transitional arrangements do not affect any midwife who has registered as a midwife after April 1995. She will need to meet the PREP study requirements in the same way as any other registrant.

The key points to remember are (UKCC 1997b):

• Midwives refresher courses will continue to be valid for practising midwives until superseded by the full PREP requirements in April 2001.

• Practising midwives do not need to undertake the study requirements of PREP *in addition* to their refresher course requirements.

• When the PREP rules are fully operational for midwives, it will mean 5 days of updating every 3 years, instead of a 5 day course or accumulated study days every 5 years.

- The PREP study activity requirements do *not* require approval in the way refresher courses have done. As the PREP study activity requirements supersede the current refresher course requirements for midwives, the need for National Board courses of study activity will gradually be phased out. It will be a matter for the National Boards in each country of the UK to decide when this will occur. Return to practice courses will, however, continue to require approval by a National Board.
- Practising midwives will continue to notify their intention to practice annually *in addition* to completing their notification of practice form every 3 years when re-registering with the UKCC.

The programmes

The programmes must be approved by a National Board for Nursing, Midwifery and Health Visiting. They must be no less than 5 days in length. No maximum time is in place, in order to allow for individual needs and abilities. Programmes should be as flexible as possible to meet the needs of the returning nurse, midwife and health visitor, the length being decided by the individual and the education provider. The individual's registration, their previous experience and knowledge and any relevant experience obtained whilst out of practice will all help to decide the length and nature of the programme. Whatever the final 'shape' of the programme, the following *outcomes* must be met (UKCC 1996b):

- an understanding of the influence of health and social policy relevant to the practice of nursing, midwifery and health visiting
- an understanding of the requirements of legislation, guidelines, codes of practice and policies relevant to the practice of nursing, midwifery and health visiting
- an understanding of the current structure and organization of care, nationally and locally
- an understanding of the current issues in nursing, midwifery and health visiting practice
- the use of relevant literature and research to inform the practice of nursing, midwifery and health visiting
- the ability to identify and assess need, design and implement interventions and evaluate outcomes in all relevant areas of practice, including the effective delivery of appropriate emergency care
- the ability to use appropriate communications, teaching and learning skills
- the ability to function effectively in a team and participate in a multiprofessional approach to the care of patients and clients
- the ability to identify strengths and weaknesses, acknowledge limitations of competence and recognize the importance of maintaining and developing professional competence.

BEING REGISTERED

The PREP legislation substantially changes the nature of registration. Before 1 April 1995, all individuals who had ever been registered with the UKCC or one of its predecessor bodies – the General Nursing Council for England and Wales, the General Nursing Council for Scotland, the Central Midwives Board for England and Wales, the Central Midwives Board for Scotland, the Northern Ireland Council for Nurses and Midwives, the Council for the Education and Training of Health Visitors, the Panel of Assessors for District Nurse Training, the Joint Board for Clinical Nursing Studies and the Committee for Clinical Nursing Studies (Scotland) – stayed registered regardless of what else happened. The only way an individual could lose their registration was if it was taken away by the UKCC's professional conduct committee. An individual's registration was either 'effective' – which meant that you had paid your fee on a 3-yearly basis (and for midwives, met the Rule 37 requirements) – or 'ineffective', which meant that you had not paid your fee. An effective registration was needed to practise as a nurse, midwife or health visitor.

This all changed with PREP. Your registration is now, in effect, your licence to practise. Either the requirements *are* met for registration or your registration lapses. Once lapsed, your registration as a 'licence to practice' has the same value as a lapsed insurance policy – in other words, none. This seems rather harsh written down like this, but it is a matter of fact and it is important that it is understood. At the risk of restating the obvious, you *must* be registered with the UKCC to be employed as a registered nurse, midwife or health visitor. Employers are increasingly taking a hard line with those individuals whose registration has been found to have lapsed, for whatever reason. Sanctions can range from immediate suspension without pay, to suspension with pay, to being replaced or shadowed by a registered practitioner and being paid as an auxiliary until registration is renewed. All very unpleasant, expensive and quite unnecessary. Ensuring that your registration is effective is *your* responsibility. The date is on your PIN card and the UKCC remind you of the expiry of your registration – provided you have given them your current address. However, employers also have a responsibility and they should have effective personnel systems in place to ensure that everyone is registered and to remind individuals as the time approaches (UKCC 1995c).

You do, of course, retain your *qualification*, regardless of circumstances – like any other qualification, once obtained it is yours for life. It is the concept of registration as a licence to practice which has changed so significantly.

Renewing registration

In case you are now racked with guilt about your own lapsed registration, let's look at what you have to do to renew it. If your registration has been lapsed for less than 3 months, then you merely have to write, phone or e-mail the registrations department of the UKCC requesting re-registration, paying your fee and completing your notification of practice form. If it has been lapsed for longer than 3 months, then you are obliged by law to provide three references supporting your application. This is to reduce the possibility of anyone committing any offence whilst unregistered, which may mean that they are not suitable for re-registration, without the UKCC being fully aware of the circumstances. It will also be necessary to make good any deficits in study requirements before re-registering. Whatever else you do, don't freeze with panic and do nothing – that's the worst thing you can do.

Use of the title registered nurse, midwife or health visitor

As you would imagine, one of the things that was of considerable concern to many of those already on the register was the potential loss of a very valued title. Many people are rightly very proud of their state registered nurse (SRN) or state certified midwife (SCM) title and did not want to lose it. As PREP is about ensuring that those currently practising maintain professional knowledge and competence – not about gratuitously offending everyone who has given sterling service to their profession in the past – the following position was agreed (UKCC 1994b).

Where an individual's registration has lapsed, the individual nurse, midwife or health visitor must ensure the he/she does not imply, directly or indirectly, that he/she is registered with the UKCC. Reference to qualifications described by the use of letters, such as SRN, SCM, RGN or RM, may be acceptable, for example, for private correspondence purposes. They cannot, however, actually or by implication, be used for the purposes of securing or continuing in a role requiring registration with the UKCC when the individual in question is not actually registered. This is the case regardless of whether the individual is in a paid position or not. It is an offence under Section 13 of The Nurses, Midwives and Health Visitors Act 1997 to intend 'to deceive'.

CONCLUSION

I hope that this chapter has been helpful in reminding you of the actual PREP requirements. They are not onerous, but neither are they to be taken lightly. The requirements were put into place for a purpose – to help individuals to maintain and develop their professional knowledge and competence. This is a serious business and one which we all have to honour, as part of our personal professional accountability and our wish to serve the public for whom we care.

REFERENCES

Cerevo R 1988 Effective Continuing education for professionals. Jossey Bass, San Francisco

Dilloway M, Garbett R, Bagnell P 1997 Nurses' experiences of continuing education. Nursing Times 25: 48–50

HMSO 1993 The Welsh Language Act. HMSO, London

HMSO 1995 The Nurses, Midwives and Health Visitors (Periodic Registration) Rules Amendment Order 1995 SI 967. HMSO, London

Kolb DA 1984 Experiential learning. Prentice Hall, New Jersey

Lauder W 1994 Beyond reflection: practical wisdom and the practical syllogism. Nurse Education Today 14: 91–98

Schon D 1983 Understanding the need for artistry in professional education in educating the reflective practitioner. Basic Books, New York

Schon D 1987 Educating the reflective practitioner. Jossey Bass, London

The Stationery Office 1997 The Nurses, Midwives and Health Visitors Act 1997. The Stationery Office, London

UKCC 1993a Midwives rules. UKCC, London

UKCC 1993b Registrar's letter 1/1993. The council's position concerning a period of support and preceptorship. UKCC, London

UKCC 1994a PREP fact sheets. UKCC, London (out of print)

UKCC 1994b The future of professional practice – the council's standards for education and practice following registration (PREP) – position statement (number 1), 1 March 1994. UKCC, London

UKCC 1995a Registrar's letter 3/1995. The council's position concerning a period of support and preceptorship. UKCC, London

UKCC 1995b Registrar's letter 19/1995. The council's standards for education and practice following registration – return to practice programmes. UKCC, London

UKCC 1995c Registrar's letter 15/1995. PREP, professional conduct and lapsed registration. UKCC, London

UKCC 1996a Registrar's letter 17/1996. The future of professional practice following registration (PREP) – recognition of unwaged experience. UKCC, London

UKCC 1996b Registrar's letter 7/1996. The council's standards for education and practice following registration – return to practice programmes. UKCC, London

UKCC 1997a PREP and you. UKCC, London

UKCC 1997b Midwives refresher courses and PREP. UKCC, London

7

Specialist and advanced practice, CATS and APEL

The opera ain't over 'til the fat lady sings.

(Dan Cook)

INTRODUCTION

This chapter looks at two separate, but related, issues. Firstly, it looks at the specific requirements, where they exist, relating to specialist and advanced practice. It also describes the detail of the specialist practice qualification Secondly, it looks at the issue which is so important if you are thinking of doing further study and acquiring further qualifications – that of the recognition and accumulation of credit for previous learning, whether that learning has been by means of taught courses or from experience.

SPECIALIST AND ADVANCED PRACTICE

In their review of specialist and advanced practice, Wallace & Gough (1995) commented that the debate over specialist and advanced practitioners 'has had a long and tortuous history'. Writing at the very end of 1997, little seems to have changed. As has already been made clear in earlier parts of the book, the discussions on specialist and advanced practice were the ones that caused the greatest challenge. The trouble was that everyone who took part in the debate had an answer – it was just that they were all different!

This part of the work had by far the longest and most convoluted history – which probably goes some way to explaining why it was so difficult to resolve. Indeed, it was put to me early on in the debates, that if something had been talked about for that many years, without a satisfactory solution being found, it was probably because it was actually insoluble – certainly in terms of finding a solution with which all the interested parties would be content.

You may remember that Project 2000 (UKCC 1986) had left the debate at the point of three recommendations relating to the 'specialist practitioner', as follows:

- *Recommendation 11*. There should be specialist practitioners, some of whom will also be team leaders, in all areas of practice in hospital and community settings. The requisite qualifications will be recordable on the UKCC's register.
- *Recommendation 12*. Health visiting, occupational health nursing and school nursing should be specialist qualifications in health promotion which are recordable on the UKCC's register.
- *Recommendation 13*. District nursing, community psychiatric nursing and community mental health nursing should be qualifications that are recordable on the UKCC's register.

In essence, Project 2000 proposed that there be two main categories of specialist practitioners: those concerned with health promotion of the well population and those concerned with clinical specialties.

This is where the PREPP project took up the story. The debates and discussions which took place during the early days of the project are well rehearsed in Chapter 5 and will not be repeated here. Suffice it to say that after all the heart-searching, passionate debates, arguments, dissensions and compromises, a conclusion was finally reached. Let us now look at the final result.

Midwives

After much debate, midwives finally decided that specialist practice was not appropriate for, or relevant to, midwifery practice. The integrated nature of the midwifery service requires education as a midwife to prepare individuals to give safe and effective care in all settings. Any changes to a midwife's role, to accommodate changes in care delivery, are subsequently incorporated into the initial preparation leading to registration. Similarly, post-registration activity is influenced by the integrated nature of the midwifery service, with more of an emphasis on keeping up-to-date through 'refresher' activity than on the acquisition of specific skills through post-registration courses. It was recognized, however, that there would be many practitioners who would wish to undertake professional development in addition to the statutory minimum of 5 days of study activity and should be encouraged to do so.

What follows next, therefore, in relation to specialist qualifications relates in the main to nursing, although there will, of course, be some midwives who will undertake specialist programmes suitable for midwives or nurses, in some areas of care, such as neonatal care.

Specialist nursing practice

It was certainly not envisaged that every registered nurse needs a specialist qualification. The UKCC recognized that clinical and caring teams will change in their composition over time, in order to adjust to changing demands, in terms of knowledge, skills and the organization of care delivery. Teams will therefore require individuals with a range of knowledge and experience. For many individuals, the knowledge that is acquired during their pre-registration preparation, the regular updating required by PREP, together with all the knowledge and experience obtained through the actual practice of their profession, will be sufficient to meet both their own professional needs and, more importantly, the needs of those for whom they care. This is an important point and one on which practitioners need to be clear and secure in their information. The standards for specialist practice have been agreed for those in, or wishing to achieve, positions requiring additional knowledge and skills. It is also important to be clear that it is not a requirement of the UKCC that everyone working in a particular area of practice, where specialist qualifications are available, must have such a qualification.

The value of the new specialist qualifications will only be proven over time and their success will lie, in large part, with how valuable employers see it to be. The criteria for success, understandably, is likely to be the 'added value' element. In other words, what is there about this individual, who has completed expensive additional training, that will mean that the trust's/nursing home's/general practice's business will be done more effectively and efficiently? How do such individuals compare to someone who has not done a similar additional programme?

So, what has actually been said about specialist practice? I quote in full from *The Future of Professional Practice – the Council's Standards for Education and Practice following Registration* (UKCC 1994a):

Whilst pre-registration education provides practitioners with the knowledge, skills and attitudes to give safe and effective care, professional practice alone following registration is not enough to meet additional specialist needs. Specialist health care and specialist patient/client requirements call for additional education for safe and effective practice. There is, therefore, a need for some practitioners to be able to exercise higher levels of judgment and discretion in clinical care to function as specialist nursing practitioners. Such specialist practitioners will demonstrate higher levels of clinical decision making and will be able to monitor and improve standards of care through supervision of practice, clinical nursing audit, developing and leading practice, contributing to research, teaching and supporting professional colleagues.

So far, so good. The key question, however, was: where were these areas of practice in which specialist practitioners might work? The answer was that it could be anywhere, in any field of professional practice, where there was an additional body of knowledge and skill that could enhance patient and client care. The UKCC only specified the eight areas of practice within the community where specialist qualifications would be available because that was what had been asked for during the consultation on the community education and practice project, described in Chapter 5. However, it was decided not to specify areas of specialist practice in the sector, often rather clumsily and increasingly inappropriately referred to as the 'institutional' sector. This was an intentional decision to allow for maximum flexibility and responsiveness, so that changes in care delivery and knowledge could be accommodated over time. Provided that the programmes met the general and specific criteria set out below, and the course was approved by a National Board for Nursing, Midwifery and Health Visiting, then specialist preparation could be available to meet demand, in all areas of nursing practice.

Specialist qualifications

The content of programmes leading to a specialist qualification, which prepare practitioners for specialist nursing practice, comprise four broad areas:

- clinical nursing practice
- care and programme management
- clinical practice development
- clinical practice leadership.

Let us look at these each in turn.

Clinical nursing practice. This is probably the most obvious area of content. It will deal with the practice-specific knowledge and skill relevant to the area in which the individual is working. It does, however, recognize that *all* areas of nursing practice have their special skills and knowledge. Good examples are general medical/surgical nursing, which had in the past rather lost out, in terms of specific preparation, to the more 'glamorous' areas traditionally associated with 'specialist courses' such as intensive care or renal nursing.

This element of the programme, if it is separately packaged, may well be the one that individuals will complete first, if they undertake the qualification on a modular basis, as it is the one which is most specifically focused on improving safe and effective practice. It may indeed be the case that this is the element for which employers would provide full support, as it has such obvious and direct effect on patient/client care.

Care and programme management. This part of the programme relates to the individual patient/client, the family, the community and the environment of care. The individual will gain additional knowledge in relation to drawing together the relevant agencies in hospital and the community which are needed to deliver care more effectively. Focusing on direct care and the promotion of health and on disease prevention, it will also emphasize the importance of actively detecting problems, risks and needs, and not merely responding to stated demand.

Clinical practice development. This element of the programme will concentrate on the acquisition of skills needed to give an ever-improving quality of service, including the monitoring, evaluating and auditing of standards. An in-depth knowledge of clinical practice development, particularly in the practitioner's own area of practice – together with related areas – will be acquired, helping the individual to apply the new developments to their field of practice, where relevant, and to devise new approaches to care. Individuals will also acquire a detailed knowledge of relevant research relating to their area of practice and how it can best be applied.

Clinical practice leadership. This is the element of the programme which will prepare the practitioner to lead, support and supervise others in professional practice and their support staff, oversee students' practice placements, to ensure that best use is made of them and to ensure staff development and provide practice-based teaching.

Academic standards for the programmes

In order to be approved by a National Board, programmes leading to a specialist qualification (SQ) must meet the following criteria. They must have clearly defined outcomes and be:

- an academic year in length (no less than 32 weeks)
- no less than first degree level study (see below)
- modular, where possible
- flexible
- accessible full- or part-time
- approved by a National Board
- arranged around a common core framework with specialist modules
- linked to a higher education accreditation system, with credit being given for appropriate prior learning and appropriate experiential learning.

The only exception to this standard was that for the period of the transitional arrangements (see pp 142–143), in areas of practice where no previous recordable qualifications were available, programmes could be approved at diploma level. This was to ensure that those practitioners for whom no qualifications in their area of practice had been previously available were not disadvantaged by having to take too large an academic ' jump' between their pre-registration qualification and their specialist qualification (UKCC 1995).

Programmes leading to a specialist qualification are available for all those on the professional register. Second level (enrolled) nurses also need to have reached the outcomes for first level registration by the time of completing a specialist qualification, so that they will be eligible to register as a first level nurse, at the same time as recording their specialist qualification.

Community specialist practice

The following areas for which a specialist qualification will be available in the community are (UKCC 1991):

- general practice nursing
- community children's nursing
- community mental handicap (now known as learning disabilities) nursing
- community mental health nursing
- public health nursing/health visiting
- occupational health nursing
- nursing in the home/district nursing
- school nursing.

All programmes leading to qualifications in the above areas must meet the standards for specialist qualifications.

Transitional arrangements

Given that whole of the PREP consultation process had been premised on the understanding that maximum credit would be offered, where possible, to those already in practice, it was necessary to put some form of transitional arrangements into place, for those who were already 'in the system'. As with all compromise arrangements of this nature, they are rarely perfect and cannot please everyone. This was certainly the case with the PREP transitional arrangements. However, they did allow recognition of previous learning and experience for a considerable number of practitioners who would not have been so recognized, if the 'cleanest' solution had been used. This would have been to instigate an absolute cut-off between the 'old' system of recording qualifications and the provision of the 'new' specialist qualifications.

Basically, what the UKCC, together with the National Boards, agreed was an arrangement whereby those falling into the following categories could be employed in specialist practice posts and would not be required by the UKCC to undertake additional study:

- individuals who have a post-registration clinical recordable qualification of 4 months or more in length (including all school nursing programmes) relevant to their area of practice
- the individual and their employer are confident that the practitioner has the necessary skills and knowledge safely and effectively to fulfil their role as defined in the UKCC's document *The Scope of Professional Practice*.

Under these circumstances such individuals can use the title specialist practitioner. No new or additional certification will be offered by the UKCC. Individuals are reminded that they may need to undertake additional study if they do not have a qualification relevant to their area of practice, or if their qualification was acquired a long time ago and has not since been consolidated by appropriate experience (UKCC 1996).

In addition, it was agreed that the National Boards will continue to provide courses during the transitional period which could be recorded with the UKCC. These may well be in areas where recordable qualifications have not previously been available. Although such qualifications will not be specialist qualifications, they could be credited towards them, should the individual decide in due course that they wish to acquire one. Following the acquisition of such a qualification, the individual concerned may well be eligible to use the title of specialist practitioner, if they meet the criteria set out above.

Advanced practice

As you will have already read, the concept of advanced practice was one which caused considerable discussion and debate, with strongly polarized positions being adopted by many of those involved. At the stage of agreeing its general position on a framework for post-registration and practice, in March 1994, the UKCC decided not to go ahead with setting standards for advanced practice. It did, however, adopt a position which committed it to exploring and developing the concept of advanced practice. Advanced practice was described as an important field of professional practice concerned with the continuing development of professionals in the interests of patients, clients and the health services. It was also at pains to stress that advanced practice was not an additional layer of practice to be added to specialist practice. The following statements were issued and also reiterated in PREP fact sheet 7 (UKCC 1994b):

Advanced midwifery practice was described as being concerned with:

- adjusting the boundaries for the development of future practice
- advancing clinical practice, research and education to enrich midwifery practice as a whole
- contributing to health policy and management and the determination of health needs
- continuing the development of midwifery in the interests of the mother, the baby, and the health service.

It was thought that advancing midwifery practice in this way would lead to:

- innovations in practice
- an increase in midwifery research and research-based practice
- the provision of expert professionals who will have a consultancy role
- high level professional leadership
- increased political and professional influence in respect of the development of maternity services
- expert resources for, for example, education, supervision, management.

Advanced nursing practice was described as being concerned with:

- adjusting the boundaries for the development of future practice
- pioneering and developing new roles which are responsive to changing needs
- advancing clinical practice, research and education to enrich nursing practice as a whole
- contributing to health policy and management and the determination of health needs
- continuing the development of the profession in the interests of patients, clients and the health services.

It was thought that advancing nursing practice in this way would lead to:

- innovations in practice
- an increase in nursing research
- the provision of expert professionals who will have a consultancy role
- high level professional leadership
- increased political and professional influence in respect of nursing and health services
- expert resources for, for example, education, supervision, management.

During 1994 and 1995, the UKCC continued to monitor progress in relation to advanced practice in both nursing and midwifery. Examples of advanced practice were examined and discussions were held with a wide range of individuals with an interest in the subject, e.g. providers of courses in 'advanced practice', practitioners who were employed in 'advanced practitioner roles', or employers seeking to expand the range of skills available within their workforce. It was also becoming increasingly clear that the use of the title 'nurse practitioner' needed clarification and resolution. What was clear from the great range of activity and the differing views being expressed was that further work needed to be done on acquiring a better understanding of the nature of advanced practice before this outstanding element of the PREP work could be finalized.

In order to move this debate forward, in 1996, under the guidance of an external consultant, more work was done on advanced practice. At the end of the process, in the paper prepared for the UKCC Council meeting in March 1997 (UKCC Council paper CC/97/06, unpublished), Abigail Masterson, the independent consultant who had been working with the Council on these issues, summed up as follows. Changes occurring in the delivery of health care in order to meet the demands for a healthy population were having a significant effect on the debate and needed to be taken into consideration, particularly in relation to the increasing blurring of the traditional boundaries between health and social care. Practice development, local service needs and national policy objectives were also throwing the old boundaries between professional roles and responsibilities into a state of flux.

Such changes were providing both excellent examples of innovative and exciting practice, but also significant challenges in relation to professional accountability and relationships between varying groups of health care professionals. Concern was being expressed on a number of fronts that the plethora of roles, titles and responsibilities in health care were proving confusing to consumers, employers and practitioners alike.

Initially, the work on advanced practice had been informed by an extensive literature search, which was carried out 'to identify what clarity of understanding of the terminology existed, to review the various nurse practitioner roles and consider cross-cultural comparisons' (Council paper CC/97/06). A 'listening' exercise was then carried out with a series of colloquia, written submissions, telephone interviews and face-to-face interviews with interested parties, both within nursing, midwifery and health visiting and also with other health care professionals, purchasers and providers. The views of at least 300 people were obtained during this stage. A seminar was also held with representatives of the National Boards. The activity culminated in a consultative conference in October 1996 with an invited audience of around 100 key players, to test out the views gained and the opinions expressed during the earlier part of the work.

There were a number of issues identified as a result of this activity, specifically:

- the confusion around roles, titles and responsibilities
- agreement that advanced practice was not about tasks but about a broader concept of practice, particularly advancing the practice of others
- nurse practitioner models based on the degree level education and assessment of practice competence were more akin to the UKCC's descriptor of specialist practice than advanced practice

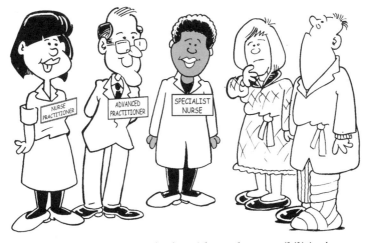

'... confusion around roles, titles and responsibilities.'

- specialist practice needed to be reconsidered in terms of how it could accommodate nurse practitioners and clinical nurse specialists
- strong support for *not* setting standards for advanced practice.

At its meeting in March 1997, the UKCC considered the results of the above activity and adopted the following position. It was decided that the UKCC, whilst fully supporting the notion of advancing practice, should not set standards for qualifications in this field. It would continue to support the concept of all practitioners advancing their practice but did not wish to pursue the idea of labelling a particular activity, or group of activities, as advanced. Further work would be done on looking at how nurse practitioners and clinical nurse specialists could be accommodated within the concepts of specialist practitioners.

To this end, a working group was established in the summer of 1997 to explore these issues in more detail, and at the time of writing the work is still being taken forward, with no prospect of an immediate solution.

My personal prediction – and I hope that I'm wrong – is that this is an issue which will never be satisfactorily resolved. I have to admit to some considerable sympathy with Colleen Wedderburn Tate, an independent nurse and health care researcher, writing in the *Nursing Standard*, who when asked to predict what will have the biggest impact on nursing in the millennium, wryly comments (Wedderburn Tate 1997):

I predict that in the year 2000 the nursing spin doctors will be meeting regularly for deep and meaningful discussions to decide what to call the latest super-advanced advanced-specialist super-duper nurse practitioner.

As an ex-spin doctor, I'd put money on it!

CREDIT ACCUMULATION AND TRANSFER/ ACCREDITATION OF PRIOR (EXPERIENTIAL) LEARNING

Let us now turn to the second part of this chapter, to consider an issue which is very relevant if you are thinking of acquiring additional qualifications – that of credit accumulation and transfer and the assessment of previous learning. These issues are particularly relevant for the practice-based professions such as nursing and midwifery, where practitioners have often accumulated vast amounts of additional knowledge and skill over time, through the process of going about their daily work – not to mention all the learning that comes merely from living! It is even more of an issue for many people on the register who, at the time of undertaking their original qualification as a nurse, midwife or health visitor, did not have an academic 'level' associated with their professional qualifications, unless they had also done a degree at the same time. As the numbers who have done a degree together with their professional qualification have always been small – about 15% of the register – that means that there are an awful lot of people who may not have acquired anything with an academic 'ticket', even though they may never have stopped learning. In my experience this is a source of great concern, and often resentment, among hard-working individuals who feel that they have at least the same level of knowledge and skill as those with more qualifications, yet without the credit for it. To an extent, I sympathize with such a view. However, it is only to a limited extent, as the blunt fact remains that our society uses qualifications as a form of 'currency' to demonstrate – rightly or wrongly – the level of knowledge and skill possessed by the holder of such qualifications – and, if that's the currency in use, then that's usually what you have to deal in. No-one, however, wants the tedious and time-consuming experience of repeating what they have already done before – which, regrettably, used to be an all too familiar feature of many courses. There is however, good news available – so please read on.

If you want to do further study, how do you avoid the unnecessary repetition of previous learning? Let's look at the issues of credit accumulation and transfer schemes (CATS) and the assessment of prior (experiential) learning (AP(E)L) in some detail. Understanding the principles of these systems is important, as there is a lot of misunderstanding around, which nearly always results in disappointment for the individual, who has had their hopes inappropriately raised.

Credit accumulation and transfer schemes

The principle behind any CAT scheme is that appropriate and relevant learning, wherever it occurs, should be given academic credit, providing it can be assessed. The original CATS was started by the now defunct Council for National Academic Awards (CNAA), but the principles have now been widely adopted throughout the higher education sector. Although probably still more sophisticated in the 'old polytechnic' sector, other more 'traditional' institutions are catching up fast. It is important to understand, however, that the choice of CAT scheme and its implementation remain the choice of the individual institution of higher education. Despite moves by the Higher Education Quality Council to streamline the approach from institution to institution, there is no national CAT scheme. Individual institutions value their autonomy too much. As a result, you may well find that different places will, to an extent, be prepared to offer different rates of credit for the same amount of previous study. This is, of course, good news and bad news. If you have the time and energy to shop around, then you may find your endeavours are rewarded, in terms of the award of maximum credit.

Let us look in more depth at CATS. The intention of the whole activity was to design a 'scheme whereby qualifications, part qualifications and learning experiences are given appropriate recognition or credit to enable students to progress their studies without necessarily having to repeat materials or levels of study' (Toyne 1979).

The whole scheme is based around the acquisition of credit points, which can be 'general' or 'specific'. 'General' credit, as its name implies, relates to an individual's general level knowledge and ability, whereas 'specific' credit relates directly to the course on which they are wishing to embark. The basic benchmark is the honours degree, for which 360 credit points are required (which will be a mixture of general and specific). A master's degree needs 120 credits at M level. The system is different in Scotland, under the SCOTCATS scheme, as the basic degree is 4 years in length. The principles, however, are the same.

Let's look at the system in more detail. The acronym gives us the necessary guidance:

C for CREDIT. This is what an individual is trying to accumulate, in points, in pursuit of a specific qualification. CATS schemes are not free-standing. In other words, you can't just acquire a random selection of 360 unrelated CATS points from various sources and call them a degree.

A for ACCUMULATION. This is how your credit points add up. Different modules of a flexible pathway degree or diploma, for example, will attach specific credit points to each module. The student will probably have to do some core (or essential) modules and then will be able to choose from a selection of other modules, providing the total points awarded add up to that required for the qualification being sought.

T for TRANSFER. Flexibility here is the key. The student should be able to take credits already acquired 'with' them, if they want to move. The move could be within the same institution, to a different course. Alternatively, it could be to another part of the UK, or indeed, even more widely. Within Europe, for example, there is a European-wide credit scheme known as ECTIS. Regardless of the nature of the specific scheme, the principle being applied is always the same – that of not having to repeat previous learning.

S for SCHEME(S). I think this is self-evident.

So far, so good. But, as always, it does get a bit more complicated in practice.

Accreditation of prior (experiential) learning

Let's also have a look at the assessment of prior learning, known as APEL, which is always associated with CATS. This relates to the process whereby you actually have your previous learning assessed, in order to accumulate the necessary credit points, for a particular CATS scheme. You can claim credit for a variety of previous learning activities, which fall broadly into two categories. Firstly, there is the learning associated with prior education, e.g. formal or certificated learning, short courses or vocational study. This is known as the assessment of prior learning (APL). Secondly, there is the assessment of the type of learning that comes from experience. This is known as the assessment of prior experiential learning (APEL). This includes the sort

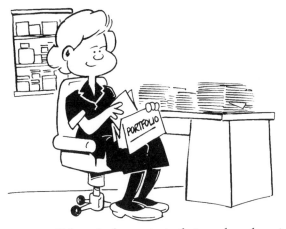

'... of course, you will have to demonstrate that you have learnt something from these experiences ...'

of learning associated with life experiences, such as bringing up children, playing sport, running the local playgroup, voluntary work, retraining after redundancy, organizing the local rugby club and so on. Experiential learning is often mistyped as 'experimental' learning, which, when you think about it, may not be so far off the mark. As you would imagine, it is easier to assess the former, rather than the latter.

But, of course, you will have to be able to *demonstrate* that you have learnt something from these experiences. Understandably, no-one is merely going to take your word for what you have done, without some form of corroboration. Each institution will have different methods whereby you can claim credit. Some, for example, will ask you to provide a portfolio of previous work. This could include things like case histories that you have previously prepared or articles you may have written. Writing essays is also a way of demonstrating your levels of previous achievement. Some institutions are also developing interactive computer programs that take you step by step through the process of claiming credit.

What are you actually claiming credit for? Remember, CAT / APEL schemes do not exist in isolation. They are about the accumulation of credit towards a specific target – this can be either credit against the entrance requirements to a particular course or credit against part of the content of the course itself. Let's look at that in a bit more detail.

Suppose you want to do a Master's degree. When you get the course information, it may tell you that entrance is 'normally' by means of a good honours degree. And as lots of people won't have a first degree, it is easy to be put off at this stage. But – many individuals will have done a lot of additional study since they first qualified. The learning acquired from this type of activity may well allow you to enter the course, following some sort of assessment. This may involve an interview, producing either previous written work or something new.

Don't be put off by the thought of such an assessment and having to do something like this. You will probably find that much to your surprise you really enjoy the process. After all, adult learning is about finding out what you *can do* – not about exposing what you *don't know*. If you haven't studied for a while, this may come as a very pleasant shock! The sort of credit that you would be awarded here will be of a general nature, because by and large what is being assessed is your general level of competence. This would include, for example, an assessment of your ability to write coherently and to marshall an argument. Even if you are not completely successful at the first attempt, which is quite likely as this may well be a completely new experience for you, don't be put off. There is likely to be a considerable amount of help at hand in the higher education institution which is designed to assist you in the process.

The other sort of credit that you may be claiming relates specifically to the particular course you want to do. For example, if you have already studied a subject to a similar level and depth of one of the course components of a specialist practice qualification, then you may be given credit, i.e. exemption, for a whole module, so that you don't have to repeat previous learning.

In terms of claiming credit, Hull & Redfern (1996) identified the following criteria against which a learning profile will be assessed. The criteria are, however, transferable across any form of credit bid, in whatever form it is presented:

- *breadth* – the learning is not isolated from other considerations
- *authenticity* – you can do what is claimed
- *quality* – the learning is at the appropriate academic level
- *currency* – you have kept up-to-date with recent developments
- *acceptability* – the evidence supports the learning claim to which it is linked
- *sufficiency* – there is enough evidence to show sufficient proof of confidence.

You will have realized by now that effective credit schemes require a number of things to be successful. First, and probably most importantly, you need an institution that is really signed up to the philosophy of credit. Second, you probably need modular provision of the courses. It is difficult to manage effective credit on a linear course, i.e. one which starts on 1 September and goes straight through a taught course without a break, except for holidays, with all students doing the same thing. The flexibility of provision which goes with modular courses does make it easier to manage a good credit system.

Do remember, however, that each individual institution will have their own internal requirements for credit. For example, some, in order to ensure the internal coherence of course and to avoid fragmentation and lack of cohesion, will only award credit up to a certain maximum, however much previous learning an individual has undertaken. In some institutions, at least 75% of the course must be taught, but it can be a lot lower than that.

CONCLUSION

This chapter has been a continuation of the previous one, to an extent, but has concentrated on the aspects of the PREP requirements which have been most complex and difficult to resolve, i.e. specialist and advanced practice and the associated qualifications. I have also chosen, I think appropriately, to look at the detail of claiming credit, which is very relevant to the acquisition of additional qualifications. Having now looked the context, the background and the PREP requirements themselves, it is necessary to start to apply this knowledge and see what this all means for *you*, as one of the individuals concerned.

REFERENCES

HEQC 1994 Choosing to change. The report of the HEQC CAT development project. HEQC Publications, London
Hull C, Redfern L 1996 Profiles and profiling. A guide for nurses and midwives. Macmillan, London
Toyne P Educational credit transfer: feasibility study. DES, London
UKCC 1986 Project 2000: a new preparation for practice. UKCC, London
UKCC 1991 The report on community education and practice. UKCC, London
UKCC 1994 The future of professional practice – the council's standards for education and practice following registration. UKCC, London
UKCC 1994 PREP fact sheets. UKCC, London (out of print)
UKCC 1995 Registrar's letter 9/1995. The council's standards for education and practice following registration (PREP): academic level of programmes of education leading to the qualification of specialist practitioner, in the transitional period. UKCC, London
UKCC 1996 Registrar's letter 15/1996. The council's standards for education and practice following registration (PREP): transitional arrangements – specialist practitioner title/specialist qualification. UKCC, London
Wallace M J, Gough P J 1995 The UKCC's criteria for specialist and advanced nursing practice. British Journal of Specialist Nursing 1(3): 939–943
Wedderburn Tate C 1997 Nurse 2000. Nursing Standard 12(1): 24

8

Next steps

Learning is a process of discovery and we must each be our own discoverer – others cannot do it for you.

(John Dewey)

INTRODUCTION

Well, this is the last chapter, apart from the appendices. I hope that you have found the book interesting and helpful, so far. But, to a large extent, it has been someone else's story up to now. This chapter is where we start turning it into *your* story. So far, we have looked at PREP in the context of lifelong learning and continuous professional development, in terms of its own unique history and development, and also in terms of the actual requirements. All this is important stuff, but it probably feels very general and still slightly remote, although hopefully less general and less remote than when you started. Of course, you do have to be sure of your facts and by now you will be a lot more confident about what it's all about. But now comes the really important bit – what does this actually mean for *you* in your day-to-day professional and personal life? Generalities and policies are all very well, but at some stage, if you haven't done so already, you will have to sit down and consider – or reconsider – the real impact of PREP, lifelong learning and the responsibilities associated with continuing professional development on your daily life.

Remind yourself again, at this stage, of Sir Ron Dearing's description of higher education in his recent report, which was referred to in the earlier chapters. *Higher Education in a Learning Society* (National Committee of Enquiry into Higher Education 1997a) describes the purpose of higher education as follows:

- to inspire and enable individuals to develop their capabilities to the highest potential throughout life, so that they grow intellectually, are well equipped for work, can contribute effectively to society and achieve personal fulfilment

- to increase knowledge and understanding for their own sake and to foster their application to the benefit of the economy and society
- to serve the needs of an adaptable, sustainable, knowledge-based economy at local, regional and national levels
- to play a major role in shaping a democratic, civilized, inclusive society.

These are stirring words and are relevant to all of us on the professional register. Even if the original education you undertook was not in higher education, the level of your subsequent knowledge and experience may well have been, and that is the level at which practice needs to operate now. The descriptors above apply to you and should frame your thoughts for the future. How do we translate those ideals into a practical, workable, affordable reality?

What this chapter does is suggest some practical ways in which you might like to move forward. Given the number of you reading the book (I hope!) and the various qualifications, ages, experiences and personal circumstances that you have accumulated between you, clearly there can be no 'prescription' that will accommodate you all. Anyway, you will have realized by now that PREP is about freedom of choice, not imposed routes and explicit requirements. The issue, too, is much wider than PREP. Of course, there is a statutory minimum that now has to be met by all those on the register. You know the details of that by now, having got this far in the book. And it may well be that because of your current combination of circumstances, doing more than the statutory minimum is just not feasible. However, if you have not systematically assessed your situation recently, you might surprise yourself, in terms of what you are capable of or what you now feel you can or would like to do. I hope, if nothing else, reading this book has helped you to think about the nature of lifelong learning and professional development in a positive way and that you have decided to incorporate it into your future planning. Until you have really explored all the possibilities, who knows to what heights you may soar? So, whatever your life plan is at the moment (and your sole objective may currently be survival), do read on. If what I say is not relevant now, it may well be that there will be time in the future when it is. The process is timeless and can be done today, next year or in 10 years – the principles will be the same.

In order to be as helpful as possible, I have chosen to pose a range of questions/issues that you might like to think about when planning your own professional development. It is not a heavily erudite dissertation on career planning in general. It is a common sense approach which you may want to think about, taking into account your own personal preferences, your professional and personal circumstances and your short- and long-term goals and aspirations.

If you have gleaned any message from your reading of this book so far, it will have been that having embarked on a process like PREP – however much the details of it may change in the future (which, of course, they are bound to, as the policies are evaluated in practice) – the idea of continually updating your knowledge and competence is here to stay. Indeed, even if PREP had not come when it did, the UKCC would be working on such a project right now – but it would be chasing behind the leaders, instead of having been in the vanguard for change.

Regrettably, the driver for such activity would probably not now be coming primarily from the need to improve professional practice, but instead from the increasing attention paid to the management of risk. The increasing emphasis on litigation and the apportioning of blame, within the context of risk management, places an increasing onus on each individual professional to not only take responsibility for their own actions, but also to be able to articulate clearly and with evidence why they adopted, for example, a particular treatment approach or manner of dealing with a specific situation.

Clinical practice, in particular, is fraught with difficulties and there appears to be little doubt that the realities of day-to-day care can be very challenging, with frequent conflicts between professional standards and the hard realities of life with insufficient staff and variable levels of managerial support. Let me give you an example that had a profound effect on me whilst writing this book. It is taken from an article in the *Nursing Times* (*Nursing Times* 1997).

It told of a junior sister on a medical ward who had had the courage and integrity (guess whose side I'm on?) to talk to a patient and his relatives about the poor prognosis associated with his recent and extensive myocardial damage following a massive myocardial infarction. Although the multi-disciplinary case conference had already decided that no resuscitation was to be carried out, no doctor had spoken to the patient or his relatives. He was seen by the nurse concerned, the next day, and found to be in need of reassurance and someone to talk to, as he was frightened and still in pain. The discussion had the effect of reassuring both the patient and his loving and anxious relatives. The next day, however, she was called in from home on her day off to explain her actions to the consultant and three managers. The managers included her own nurse manager, who said not a word in her defence. She was told in no uncertain terms that discussing prognoses with patients was the business of the doctors and no-one else. What does that sort of treatment do for the delivery of compassionate, considered nursing care and the confidence of a highly motivated and competent individual, who is endeavouring to maintain and develop her professional knowledge and competence as an accountable professional?

So, please understand that I do realize that the day-to-day realities of life are often really hard and I can quite appreciate that some people may think that PREP is just another straw designed to break the proverbial camel's back. But it's there, and will not go away. So let's see how you can make it positive, useful, relevant and – why not? – fun; something which really helps you, your patients and clients and your colleagues, in your day to day work.

ATTITUDES

I'm afraid that the next bit may sound a bit pretentious and I said at the beginning that I wanted to avoid pretentiousness at all costs.... Still, here goes, because it is important. I do think that a positive attitude to lifelong learning, professional development and PREP is really helpful, if not actually essential. Fortunately, that's what a lot of registrants do have because they can see the benefits of maintaining and developing professional knowledge and competence. If, on the other hand, you resent having to do anything at all, then the whole thing will become a real bore and you will get no benefit, and more importantly no enjoyment, out of the activity. So, that's the first thing – make up your mind that you are going to enjoy it and then you will. Reinhold Niebuhr wrote:

God grant me the serenity
To accept the things I cannot change;
The courage to change the things I can;
And the wisdom to know the difference.

This has been revamped and reproduced in a number of forms over the years – you may remember it from your management courses in a different form. Basically, it is saying don't waste time fighting the inevitable. It's the last line that's the real test though, isn't it? And probably not many of us crack that, certainly not all the time.

The next thing to realize is that the 'official' bit of PREP is, in the main, finished. Yes, more work has to be done on the audit tool and there will be changes as the policies are evaluated in practice, but the success or failure of PREP now depends on how we – the registrants – put it into practice. If you have some good ideas about implementation, write to the UKCC and tell them. You will have realized by now that policy-making is by no means an exact science and it's easy to get it wrong – or at least not as right as it may be. So good ideas are always welcome, especially when it is about the UKCC's policies in action. The Council really does want to hear about the way its requirements work in practice. In his memoirs *Conflict of Loyalties*, Geoffrey Howe (1995) comments, after the dissemination of a particular policy, and having received a letter (not from a Tory voter) congratulating him on his action: 'I wonder if those who take the trouble to write such letters realize how tremendously they add to the confidence of the recipient.' This is so true – it is a real pleasure to get letters from people commenting on policies. They don't necessarily have to be in agreement with the policies in question, although it helps – when the writer disagrees – if they say why and offer positive alternative proposals. Those who are involved in policy-

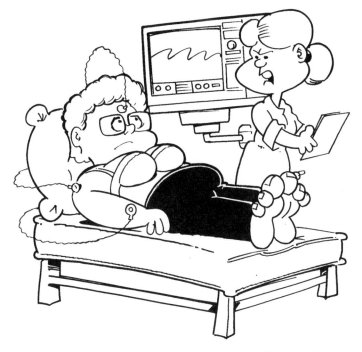

'What could have been a boring morning spent at a local hospital became much more interesting when, stripped to the waist, flat on my back and festooned with electrodes … the staff nurse started to tell me her concerns about PREP.'

making, by and large, have no illusions that what they do is perfect. I am, of course, talking about the UKCC. I have no insight into the minds of Tory politicians!

I was very cheered with a personal experience which occurred whilst I was writing this book. I had to have a medical for a World Health Organization consultancy assignment that I was doing in the Middle East and needed a chest X-ray, ECG and some bloods amongst other things. What could have been a boring morning spent at the local hospital became much more interesting, when – stripped to the waist, flat on my back and festooned in electrodes (not a pretty sight!) – the staff nurse started to tell me of her concerns about PREP. In case you wondered, I had confessed to some knowledge of the subject. Her situation, I would imagine, was not uncommon. She had been out of nursing for 14 years but had recently returned to the nurse bank, before being offered a permanent post in outpatients. She was very positive about PREP but needed reassurance that she did not have to do 'formal' study days. She was also having difficulty trying to find a return to practice course, which she had identified as something she needed for this year. The nearest one with any vacancies was in Nottingham – and we were in Berkshire at the time! Still, she was going to persevere because she thought that the whole idea was a good one and was treating the whole thing as an interesting challenge.

On the other hand, I was also rather depressed when speaking at a large nursing exhibition in London in the autumn of 1997 to hear that a speaker colleague – someone who was not a nurse herself – was accused by one of the registered nurses in her audience of using 'jargon' that people did not understand. The jargon? She had referred to the UKCC! Even when she explained what the initials stood for, the individual had not heard of the organization. Oh dear, I wonder who she has been registering with since 1983… Or worse, who has she *not* been registering with?

So, which of these practitioners are you like? It must be the former or you wouldn't have got as far as reading this book! What are *you* going to do to incorporate the PREP requirements into your busy schedule? Let's look at some options, ranging from the sublime to the ridiculous (you have to guess which is which!). First of all, though, there are a number of things that you need to think about, in relation to your own personal preferences, your own personal circumstances, your plans for the future and any other variables, both foreseeable and unforeseeable. It is worth giving these things some thought at this stage in order to help you plan realistically for any future action. What you choose to do will, in large part, depend on the answers to the questions set out below. There are, of course, no right or wrong answers to the questions – everyone will have a unique set of responses depending on their own personal circumstances.

PLANNING

Are you the sort of person that plans your career? If so, I guess that you are probably in the minority, particularly if you are a woman – and as 540 000 on the register are female, the chances are that you are. On the whole, from evidence and anecdote, it would appear that men are likely to be more single-minded about where they are going career-wise and women are more likely to take opportunities which fit in with their own personal circumstances at the time. Career patterns are, however, changing significantly as job opportunities and expectations change. So, like all generalizations, mine can be open to challenge. Fortunately for the point that I am making, that does not matter – what matters is that you recognize what sort of decision-maker you are yourself. Do you prefer things to happen to you or do you prefer to make things happen? If you haven't consciously thought about this before and you don't know the answer yet, just think back over a few of the events of your life – they don't have to be enormously significant ones – and think about how much of the action was controlled by you, or whether you were a fairly passive partner in what was happening. If your brain has seized up, try the answers to these questions:

- What made you go into nursing/midwifery?
- How do you decide where to go on holiday?
- How did you meet your current partner?
- Do you have sugar in your tea? Why?
- Why are you living where you do?
- How many children do you have? Why?
- Do you like you current job? If not, why are you still there?

Fortunately, as you will have quickly realized, there are no right and wrong answers to the questions, but if you really think about them – not merely the first superficial answer – you may surprise yourself. When I tried this, at the request of a friend who was doing some research for a master's degree, I started off with the statement that I had been fairly passive in my decision-making and that my career had been a case of 'drift' rather than 'plan'. Yet when I came to examine actual events, I realized that my own actions had significantly affected the results on every occasion. A final comment – when I mentioned this to family and friends, they all said: 'Well, that's hardly a surprise, is it? We could have told you that.' Moral: it may be well worth doing this exercise with someone else!

The point of doing this is to say that you may need to change your habits a bit, if you are going to make the best use of your time and resources. If you are not a natural planner then you will need to start acquiring the skills or you will be wasting a lot of valuable time and energy. My guess is that you probably already have many of the skills, but they may not be something that you think about very often or explicitly. You may not even realize that you do it. For example, are you the sort of person that makes a list out at the beginning of the weekend, of all that needs to be done? If so, you are already on the planning road. You may well find that you are already using these skills in relation to the day-to-day exigencies of daily living but have not necessarily thought of applying them to your own professional learning needs. It does help, however, to do it in a systematic fashion. So, what sorts of things have to be considered?

CIRCUMSTANCES

Having looked at your own decision-making style, you now need to look fairly hard at your own circumstances. Again, all fairly obvious questions once you start to think about them, but you may not have done so in any systematic way up to now. What things do you need to take into account? Let us look at the issues of time and its management, the amount and type of support you receive, the amount and type of support you need, your finances, your personal study preferences, your own abilities and your short-, medium- and long-term objectives. Once this has been done, then you will be in a very good position to decide what you are going to do next – as in tomorrow, next month, next year, 2 years hence, 10 years hence and so on. Don't put the book down yet, you might actually enjoy this – no money back if you don't, though! But you might like to write and tell me what else you'd like in the next edition.

Don't be put off by all this activity. You may well decide after a consideration of all the facts that the most you can or want to do at the moment is the minimum statutory requirements for PREP. If so, that's fine. At least you will have given the matter some thought and made your own decision. On the other hand, you may surprise yourself and you may decide that you have both the interest and the energy to embark on more substantial activity, such as a further clinical course or a degree – and, if so, you would create the necessary time.

So let's start. What needs to be considered? When I casually mentioned, some time ago now, that I would like to do a master's degree my husband's response was: 'Fine, but you go to bed at midnight, get up at 5.15 a.m. and you're out of the house at work from 6.30 to about 8 most days. When exactly did you have in mind for the study?' Actually this was a very helpful comment, which made me stop and think. I then embarked on an assessment based on the sorts of considerations set out below. You may want to consider the issues in a different order, although I hope I have set them out in a logical way.

Time

This is probably the most difficult issue of all. Where are you going to find the time to do anything extra? Your 'normal' day probably already consists of some or all of the following which need to be accommodated if you are thinking of taking on anything else.

Paid work. This could be full- or part-time. Either way is hard and physically and emotionally demanding, especially with many places having their staffing levels cut to what many observers would say are dangerously low levels in relation to patient/client comfort and safety. Remember, if you are working part-time, you may well be working 'harder' physically than those working full-time. This is merely a comment not a criticism of full-timers! It may sound strange but, if you are part-time in clinical practice then you probably do more of the necessary physical 'graft' and less of the attending of meetings, writing reports, planning etc., which can give you some sort of a break from the physical activity of care. The chances are, too, that if you have to do this additional work, it gets done in your own time.

Family commitments. Virtually everyone has family commitments of some sort or another which call upon their time, on a regular or intermittent basis. This can include the more obvious daily activities such as getting the children up, dressed, fed, watered and off to playgroup/school/college. There are also the commitments to elderly parents, whether that involves a regular weekly/monthly visit or a daily round of ensuring comfort and safety. And it is important not to forget the 'work' that goes with maintaining regular contact with the extended family – visits, phone calls, letters, birthday cards and so on. There is also the commitment to self – just getting up and out in the mornings seems to take up some people's energy quota for the day (I will apologise to my son before this goes into print!).

Friends. Not everyone has a family, but fortunately most of us have friends. To be a good friend also takes time, so don't forget to include them when considering your commitments. Good friendships, like other growing things, need nurturing and attention, in the form of letters, e-mails, phone calls, meals, visits, time to talk and, more importantly, to listen, which all take time.

Social events. If you're not too exhausted, there are all those social events to include in your time tally. Whatever turns you on – playing sport, mountaineering, clubbing, eating out, chatting with friends and family, surfing the net – all out-of-work activity that takes more time out of that rapidly diminishing day.

Voluntary work. With everything else going on, it is amazing that many people still find time to include unpaid work in their regular schedule, whether that be voluntary service with the Red Cross, Amnesty, Samaritans or Citizen's Advice Bureaux, for example, or merely washing what seems like 500 pairs of rugby socks each week!

Travel. All these activities are likely to be in different places and have to be reached – travelling from one thing to another can be a great consumer of time, especially if you don't have your own transport (which is expensive, even if convenient), and public transport is often expensive and inefficient in terms of getting you exactly where you want to go to, at the time you want to get there.

Rest. This element of one's day often does not get much of a mention, but does need to be included. We all need some sleep, although you may have already had to ask some unpalatable questions about how much (the question in reality is usually how little) sleep you need/can manage on – two different issues. Remember, Maggie Thatcher, Churchill and Napoleon used to manage on about 4 hours a night – on second thoughts, perhaps I won't pursue that one. And in more detail – does the sleep have to be all in one go, can you cat nap if necessary, or can you save some 'top-up' sleep for your days off?

Personal space. Not just jargon and not unobtainable. We all need some time that is our 'own' to do whatever we need to relax and recharge the batteries. Never look on it as a luxury but as an absolute necessity in terms of your long-term mental health and survival. You might have to double up on activity here – what about an interruption-free, long, aromatic, luxurious bath, with the phone unplugged and some music of your own choice playing?

Other things. There are probably loads of other things that you do on a daily basis that have not been included here but are part of your regular routine and take up your time – reading, praying, yoga, working out... The list is endless, but I am sure that you get the idea.

The unexpected. Always allow for it because when something does crop up you will already have put in some space for dealing with it and you can feel appropriately virtuous and not too stressed by it – and if, miraculously, nothing does crop up, then that's unexpected in its own right, so make the most of it and be pleased that you have gained yourself some precious breathing space.

Time management

Yes, I know that talking to busy people about time management is an insult but bear with me for a bit longer. You will probably have realized by now what I am getting at. If you are thinking of doing something else in the way of additional activity – be it study days, longer term qualifications or whatever – time has to be found from within your current schedule. Time is not an everlastingly elastic commodity, although you sometimes feel as though it needs to be. You may well have to make some choices here. Examine your current schedule with a very critical eye – again, this is something that may well be done better with someone else. If you have the time, why not look at it with someone who is not very involved with the detail of your personal life first, who can ask the awkward questions like 'Well, why do you do that?' or 'Why do it that way?' or 'Have you ever thought of this?' Then you need to do it again with those most closely involved with you. The sorts of questions you need to ask in order to see if you can find some additional space are:

- What can go out of your schedule, either permanently or temporarily?
- What absolutely *has* to be done?
- What absolutely has to be done by *you*?
- What could be done by others?
- What would you like to retain?
- What are you happy to drop?
- What are you prepared to drop?
- What can be put on hold until you've finished whatever you plan to do?

What support do you need?

Once again the answers to this will depend to a large extent on your own circumstances. Some people are happy organizing all the physical activity themselves, secure in the knowledge that it will then be done in the way they like it. If this is the case, the only support you will need will be psychological – supportive interest and someone to talk to. Even here, though, there will be a need for contingency support for emergencies. Others will want all the help that they can get – both physical and psychological – in order to cope with taking on anything new. Yet others will be able to manage, providing they have some additional financial support (this will be looked at in more detail later). Most of us would probably need a mixture – someone to share the physical chores, someone to offer a shoulder to cry on, or someone who could take the children, dogs or granny off our hands when an assignment is due.

Now let's look at what support is actually available, if any. It is a fact of life that a lot of people do have to manage very much on their own, at least for some periods of their life. If this is the case for you at the moment, then so be it. Your plans may have to go on hold for a while. If this is the case, there is still a lot in this chapter that will be of interest to you. Personal circumstances change and you want to be ready to meet them.

What support is available to you?

Have you considered all possible means of support to help you get things done amongst family and friends. Start within the house. Is it time for a few behavioural changes on the part of your nearest and dearest? Working the washing machine does not need an NVQ, picking up dirty clothes from round the house is not a skill legally limited to mothers, shops do sell food to those of either sex, microwaves and ovens do not make value judgments

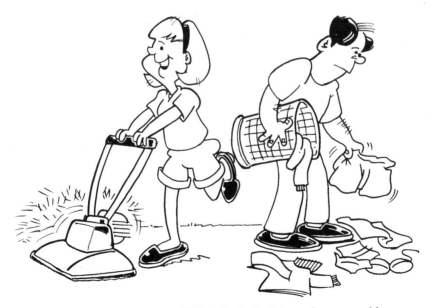

'Picking up dirty linen is not a skill legally limited to mothers … and lawns can be cut by those with an equal number of x and y chromosomes.'

about the gender of the operator and, just so that I am not accused of any bias here, cars can be serviced, washed, cleaned and maintained and lawns can be cut by those with any combination of X and Y chromosomes! Seriously, if you are embarking on something new, then your current lifestyle, and all those who contribute to it, may need some examination. This doesn't have to be a big heavy event and please don't expect to use PREP to try and secure all those behavioural changes you have been hoping for over the years (on the other hand, if it works, let me know).

Support is essential if you are going to embark on anything that will encroach into your current activity and it is much more helpful if an honest appraisal is made at the beginning – providing you err on the side of under-estimating what is available. Again, there are no right and wrong answers here. Providing the arrangements suit you and whoever else is involved then ignore the raised eyebrow, innuendos and sometimes downright rude comments you may get from other quarters. Remember, if you decide on some fairly time-consuming activity, then that is a decision to be made by all those involved, not you alone. Make sure that everyone understands what their commitment may be. For example, if you decide that you've always really wanted to do a degree, then you are not only talking about the actual taught commitment but also the reading, study and essay writing that supports it. It is quite easy to be given your space when you are physically absent – much more difficult when you can hear the hubbub of family life surging outside the door of the bedroom whilst you are trying to finish an assignment to hand in the next morning.

Do you also have the emotional support of those concerned? If not, I would suggest that you think very hard before embarking on any major activity. If, for example, 'Yes, of course. I don't mind you doing a course which will take you out two nights a week for 6 months' really means 'Yes, of course, I don't mind you doing a course…etc., etc. …providing that my meal is still available in the oven when I get home, the house stays as clean as it usually is and I can still go out with my friends on Saturday nights' then you may want to think again. We've probably all seen 'Educating Rita'! You get my drift. Don't misunderstand me, this is not an sexist, anti-partner attack; human beings of all shapes, sizes and ages can do a very good line in moral blackmail. Only *you* know what *you* are likely to face.

Fortunately, human beings can also be amazingly supportive and you may well be pleasantly surprised as everyone helps and then shares in your successes. How about doing some 'time swaps' with a friend who may also want some space for their own activities. That way you both benefit. Do you have other people that you could call on – parents, relatives, neighbours, church? The list can be quite long if you are lucky and well organized. Make sure that you always have some slack in any system for emergencies – the best laid plans can easily go awry.

What I hope that you are beginning to see is that, to some extent, you have a degree of choice over how you plan your activities. Some of you, of course, will have greater freedom than others, but we all have to make decisions depending upon our own circumstances at any given time. We all have to accept, too, that such plans, however well made, may have to change if something unexpected turns up.

Finances

One of the main things that has to be considered very early on is finances. If you have absolutely no spare money available at the moment, then the other considerations may have to take a back seat for a while. On the other hand, there can be ways of getting round what may seem, at first, an insurmountable problem.

There is no statutory funding attached to PREP activity. The UKCC is often asked why there was not money put aside to provide for 'giving registrants their PREP days'. The funding for doctors to undertake their continuing medical education (CME) is often cited as an example that nurses, midwives and health visitors should have followed. The UKCC, however, could not have made any decisions on funding because, quite simply, this was something which was outside its legislative responsibilities, and therefore something over which it had no control. The UKCC had to set the standards for post-registration education and practice. It is the work of other bodies, such as the professional organizations and trade unions, to try and persuade government to fund the activities.

So, having got that clear, where do you go for possible help with your plans? That, of course, is the key – you must have plans. You will not be able to make any sensible decisions about funding until you decide what it is you want to do. You may wish to argue that this is the wrong way round but I don't think so. To decide that you have no money and therefore – for that reason alone – you can't do anything is a bit defeatist. This may sound at odds with what I said earlier, so let's look at it in a bit more detail.

It is probably best to be frank fairly early in this debate. There are no large pots of money around waiting for thousands of nurses, midwives or health visitors to dip into. You will have to work at it. On the other hand, there are unexpected sources of funding that you may not have thought of trying, so do read on. You might get some useful ideas.

Let's start with the obvious. If you are currently in employment and what you choose for your PREP requirements is relevant to the 'business' of the organization that's paying you (which, of course, it should be) then it is reasonable to expect some help from your employer. That help could come in a number of forms. If the age of miracles is not past, then you might get funding for whatever you want to do, plus travel costs and replacements costs for whoever is doing your work whilst you are away. If you have an employer like that, be extremely grateful and let us all have their name and address (and cherish them!). Most people will be less fortunate and will have to make do with something less. What might that be? You probably should expect to get the fees paid for whatever it is you need to do. You will probably also get some contribution to travel. A lot will depend on what is in the training budget for that particular year. Good employers invest in training because it improves the workforce and gets the job done better. On the other hand, cash-strapped authorities can tend to cut the training budgets quite quickly because their reduction does not demonstrate immediate negative effects. That comes a little way down the line – often after the manager who made the decision has moved on elsewhere!

You do need to make sure when you are bidding for support that you have all your arguments marshalled as to why your employer should support you – remember you will not be the only one asking for help. Don't just sit back and wait to be offered something – it may never happen.

If you do not have an employer, but are in independent practice, then clearly you will have to find your own source of funding. Similarly, if you are not currently employed you will probably have to choose options that really do require a very small financial outlay, if any. One of the good things about PREP, of course, is that you do have the option of choosing things that really do require very little money. They may need a bit more time and ingenuity but not hard cash.

What happens if you want to do more than the statutory minimum? If you want to do a degree, you may be eligible for a grant if you have not had one before. Your local authority will be able to give you that information. Try ringing them up. You may get a pleasant surprise at how helpful they can be, if you get the right person – the trick is getting the right person, and I don't have the infallible answer to that one, I'm afraid. There are often arrangements for payment over a period of time, so that you don't have to come up-front with all the money in one go. Do shop around though – the prices of higher education courses differ phenomenally, depending on the type of degree and the institution. Master's courses, for example, can range from £800 a year to £2500 – a huge difference. Cost and quality are by no means necessarily linked, so always check what you are getting for your money.

It's probably also worth finding out whether there are any local trusts or charities who may be able to help. When our children were going through university they had money for books from a local charity that had been set up to provide tools for local apprentices. As local apprenticeships are now few and far between, the trustees wisely interpret 'books' as 'tools' for students. Who knows what you may find in your area? Your local library should be a useful source of information.

The bottom line as far as PREP is concerned, however, is that the responsibility for meeting the requirements lies with *you* – the registered nurse, midwife or health visitor. If you do get help from your employer, or indeed any source, then that's wonderful; if you don't, then you may have to modify your plans and choose something which really does not have a lot of financial cost. As far as further study goes, you may well have to put your ambitions on hold until such time as a further source of money becomes available.

Attitudes to paying for one's own study do vary across the world, depending upon the financing arrangements for the educational system in place. As many of you will know, there are a large number of countries, e.g. the United States, where 'paying your way through college' has always been the norm. The principle of paying tuition fees for higher education in the UK has also now been accepted, albeit very reluctantly, by some. Although this principle is anathema to many now, it probably won't be too long before it has become an accepted part of our society – like it or not.

Personal preferences

Another thing than needs to be taken into account at this stage in your discussions – whether with yourself or with others – is your own preferences in terms of 'study work'. What, for you, constitutes enjoyable activity and what constitutes a chore? For instance, do you like or hate reading? Would you prefer to be learning a practical skill or would you rather be adding to your theoretical knowledge, or both? Do you enjoy working through problems on your own or do you need to talk things through with another human being? If so, do you need to see them face to face or are you happy with the phone, e-mail, letter etc.? Have you tried distance learning using written materials? Would you prefer to use electronic media? Is TV your most favourite medium?

Whatever conclusions you come to – and of course these issues are matters of personal preference; there are no right or wrong answers – then they will influence how you proceed. The only comment I would make, particularly if you haven't done any studying for a long time, is to be open-minded about techniques you may not have used before, or recently. Study materials of all sorts have improved beyond recognition and you may have a pleasant surprise. So don't reject anything out of hand before you have tried it.

Your own abilities

This is quite a difficult issue. On the whole, most people underestimate what they are capable of. This is particularly true if you have had bad educational experiences in the past – which often, regrettably, means for many people that you didn't enjoy school. But times change and so, fortunately, do teaching and learning methods. If you have not done any 'studying' recently, you may be very pleasantly surprised by how things have changed for the better. Adult learning is designed to capitalize on the knowledge and experience of those taking part. It is also amazing how much easier it is to learn when what you are studying is relevant to the work you are doing at the particular moment. I think this is a really important issue. If you are studying something relevant and of interest to you (and if you are not, whose fault is that? You decided what you wanted to do) then learning becomes much less of a chore. But, like all things, it is probably best to be reasonably realistic. If you know nothing about quantum physics, it may be better to wait until you have retired to start on a course and it is probably reasonable, even then, to assume that you are unlikely to get a PhD in the subject. For me, it would be something much more mundane – anything involving numbers! In case you are interested, I have no plans to do anything involving numbers, now or at any stage ever in the future. On the other hand… who knows? That's the other thing – *never* rule out anything too definitively. Who knows how your circumstances, likes and dislikes may change, even if at this stage you feel you'd need a brain transplant to undertake certain things?

Other issues

What other things do you need to take into account? It is difficult to give them a specific heading but could include things such as:

Other people's activity. If someone else in the family is embarking on a major new commitment, like a degree, this may not be the best time for you to do the same.

Lifestyle changes. If you are about to move house, get married, get divorced (hopefully not all at the same time), think hard about the implications of that on your physical and mental health. How much can you cope with at any one time?

Work requirements. Is your job likely to change much in the foreseeable future? Will there be new professional demands on you that have to be met, in terms of new knowledge and skills? Will your job still be there in the foreseeable future, or might you have to radically rethink your own career?

Physical/mental health. Is this a good time for you health-wise? If, for any reason, it isn't, then don't add unnecessary stress to your life at this time. Wait until things have improved, if they are likely to.

Setting your objectives

So, you've now looked at the actual and potential time you have; the support you need and have available; your finances; your study preferences; and a range of other things specific to you. What's next? This is when you need to start to think more explicitly about your objectives/goals/aspirations – call them what you will. What do you want to achieve? When do you want/need to achieve it/them by? Why do you want/need to achieve it/them? You may not have ever had a chance to give things much thought. If so, don't worry – you are not alone. It is very easy to be carried along on the current of life's necessary daily activities, without ever stopping to think seriously: 'Is this really what I want to do? Where I really want to go?' But now could be the time to do just that.

An important word of warning: do try and be realistic when setting your objectives. After all you want to achieve them – so don't set yourself up to fail. Try to strike a happy medium between making them so 'soft' that they don't really offer you a challenge and so 'hard' that only a miracle will get them done. Don't necessarily expect to get it right in one go either.

If you are not immediately teeming with ideas, try to think of the things that you *have* to do, the things you *need* to do, and the things you would *like* to do. You *have*, for example, to meet your statutory PREP requirements if you are going to stay registered. You might *need* to do a short course on a particular subject because you need the new knowledge and skills to be safe in your current practice. You might *like* to do a degree because you have always wanted one but have never had the opportunity. Let us look at these in more detail.

What do you have to do?

You have to meet your PREP requirements. You now know that the statutory minimum is not very arduous and there are lots of different ways of achieving it. Appendix 3 looks at some practical examples of what individuals are doing and you may want to use some of those ideas and adapt them to your own circumstances, rather than think of something entirely new. That is often a very good way of getting started until you have the confidence to branch out and do your own thing. It's also very useful if you are totally stuck for ideas, which – let's be honest – happens to all of us at some stage in our lives.

Your decisions will be influenced by all the things that you have been thinking about earlier in this chapter. It is really important to start planning your activity at the *beginning* of every 3 year period of registration. Don't leave it until the end of that period and then have to do everything in a mad panic – that way lies potential disaster and you run the very real risk of not being able to renew your registration until you have met the requirements. That would be a considerable inconvenience and one that you can well do without.

Whatever you do, don't just do nothing and hope that it will go away. I know that there are some of you who are tempted by this option (because people have told me so) but, believe me, it is really not a runner. PREP is here to stay – the idea is too good to lose. How could one any longer justify an expensive pre-registration preparation – 3 years and several thousands of pounds, never mind all the blood, sweat and tears expended during the process – and then allow an individual to practise for years without any requirements for keeping up-to-date. Definitely not an option in the 1990s and beyond. Please don't think that people will not notice. Even disregarding the possibility of you being brought into the PREP audit scheme – and of course, you have as much chance as any other registrant of being included – you will be asked about your plans by your current employer, if you have one, or, any prospective employer. If you continue to practise without having met the requirements for registration, then your registration will lapse. Practising without registration carries severe penalties with it and would never, ever, be worth the risk.

Just to pursue this idea to the end, remember the sanctions that were set out in Chapter 6. Employers are known to respond to someone not having an up-to-date registration with a range of options which range from the draconian to the merely unpleasant – they can include suspension without pay; suspension with pay; replacement with a registered nurse/midwife whilst working and being paid as an auxiliary; being paid as an auxiliary; and dismissal. These may seem very heavy measures but they reinforce the importance attached to registration and the need for both employee and employer to have effective systems in place to ensure that registration does not lapse unknowingly. If you have deliberately done so, because you have chosen not to meet the requirements, then you really cannot expect much sympathy or support – and you certainly won't get any.

One good piece of news, however, is that the PREP legislation does allow, in justifiable circumstances, for the UKCC to grant a registrant a 6 month extension in order to meet the requirements, if there have been genuine, totally unavoidable reasons for not being able to have done so by the due date. But, please be clear, this refers only to genuinely exceptional circumstances and is certainly not intended to cover those who just haven't got their act together.

So, knowing what you have to do, how are you going to achieve it? Take into account all that you have been thinking through earlier in this chapter and make your decisions accordingly. It is worth actually writing things down unless you are very good at remembering them.

Try the following sorts of questions, if the answers don't immediately jump up and stare you in the face:

• *Am I already undertaking 5 days of study activity in a 3 year period?* Remember that you can only count the 3 year period in question. You cannot carry over additional days from the previous 3 years, or roll forward days in excess of 5 additional days into the next 3 year period. For example, if you started having to meet the requirements in September 1997, the registration period in question is September 1997–August 2000. The fact that you did 10 days of study in 1996 cannot be counted in the 1997–2000 period. Similarly, if between 1997 and 2000 you do 15 days, you cannot then roll 12 forward into the next 3 year period. I would guess, however, once you are clear about this, that you may be pleasantly surprised. A large number of those on the register already do far more than the statutory minimum. It may well be that you have never really stopped to add it all up. You can't count those things that are needed to meet other statutory requirements, e.g. Health and Safety regulations like annual lifting and fire lectures, but apart from that, there may be a lot of things that you already do that would be acceptable.

• *What's already available?* The first thing to do, if you are employed, is to find out what your employer is prepared to do to help you. Many health authorities and trusts are being very supportive of their staff in pursuit of their professional development. A lot of places are actually providing in-house study days, free of charge, often with a very reasonably priced personal professional profile available as well. Do make use of these – they serve a number of excellent purposes. They help staff to get to know each other, they give you ideas for your own further development, they can be used to improve standards throughout your place of work, they can be used as your PREP days and, as a bonus, they can be really good fun – several very good reasons for finding out what is available on site! If nothing is available, find out who you need to talk to, to get something going. After all, it is in your employer's best interest to have well-motivated, up-to-date staff who are prepared to contribute positively to the 'business' of the organization.

• *What if you are self-employed?* If you are self-employed, you will have to work a bit harder at finding out what is going on, but you already know that! Try the professional press to see what is advertised. Do you have a support group within your professional organization for those who are self-employed? If not, is it worth you starting one locally? Are you happy to do your own thing and not involve anyone else; if so, that's fine.

• *Diversity.* Remember to shop around. You certainly don't have to spend a lot of money in pursuit of the days of study activity. It is most unlikely that most individuals would be in a position to pay much from their own pockets. Many externally arranged conferences and symposia, for example, will charge anything between £200 and £400 an event and personally I wouldn't want to pay that from my own pocket, and I don't see why anyone else would want to either. If you do want to, of course, and the event meets your learning needs, and you can afford it, that's fine and it's up to you. Many of us, however, I suspect, would prefer to go for the cheaper options if possible – apart from anything else, it may mean that you can do more. There is nothing in PREP about doing more than the statutory minimum. Indeed, I'm sure that a lot of people will choose to do far more than they have to. There are lots of ways of meeting the requirements which really do cost very little money. Perhaps that's the title of the next book – *PREP on a budget* or *The rough guide to PREP.* On the other hand, perhaps not!

• *What if you really do not have time for anything else outside the house?* Have you thought about distance learning. There are some wonderful, well written interesting packages now available. They allow you to work at your own speed and at whatever time of day or night you have available. Materials can be made available in book, TV, CD-Rom or tape format, to suit all tastes and pockets. Why not share material with a friend to save cost and give you someone to talk things through with?

Having looked at what you *have* to do, let us now move on to what you *need* to do. They are not, of course, mutually exclusive. Indeed, the more match there is between what you have to do and what you need to do, the easier it will be to set your objectives.

What do you need to do?

As with everything else in this chapter, only you can answer this question and, again, it will depend on your individual circumstances. Let us take a few pertinent questions to help to focus the mind (you might find Appendix 2 helpful here, in terms of where to go for information on different courses, sources of information and so on):

- *Do you currently have a job?* If so, then is there something new coming up at work which is going to place new demands on you? This could range from learning a new clinical skill to learning how to put data into a computer – and retrieve it again! Is this a new skill for your area of practice or is it just new to you because you have not worked there before? Having decided what you are going to need, you need to think about how you will achieve it. Will it require a course? If so, is there one available locally or will you have to travel? Could you safely learn the necessary skills from working with someone who already has them for a period of time? Are there lots of you who need this new knowledge? If so, it may be worth bringing someone in from outside to help you all – that may be the cheaper option. Is it possible to get the information from some written or electronic source, or does it have to be face to face contact?

- *How secure is your job?* This is a question that needs increasingly to be asked, given the comparative insecurity of the job market. It may influence your 'Is there anything I need to do?' question, as it could affect your market-ability. Past skills and abilities may need refining, renewing or even throwing out and starting again. When did you last do a mental check that what you have to offer still has a purchaser? I know this sounds harsh and a bit jargonistic but it is a fact of life in the late (very late) 20th century and beyond – that work requirements are changing and changing significantly and are very likely to demand new knowledge and skills. If so, are you ready to meet the challenge? What might you need to learn in order to be more useful to an employer or indeed yourself? Do you have any plans for acquiring that new knowledge and skills? If not, why not?

- *Do you have any new career plans?* You may be thinking of changing the direction and focus of your career, either for personal preference or because you can see it as a boom area for the future, or for a host of other reasons. If so, there may be a range of new skills that you need. For me, most recently, the new skills that I needed were keyboard and computing ones, so that I could write and communicate round the world by the most effective means as quickly and efficiently as possible. The learning process has been most enjoyable and it is always very satisfying to crack something that you have previously admired from a distance. I now have all the enthusiasm of the new convert and suffer severe withdrawal symptoms if I am deprived of my daily 'fix' on my PC, particularly e-mail.

Right, we have looked at the 'have to' and the 'need to'. Let us now turn to the 'like to'.

What would you like to do?

To an extent, this where we enter into the 'luxury' end of your objectives, having dealt with the more mundane aspects. For working in this area, you will need to have identified enough time, and probably finances, in order for them to be realistic and achievable. This may be where you are talking about longer periods of study, leading to an academic qualification such as a first degree, master's or doctorate. Alternatively, it may be the acquisition of a new professional qualification to enter an area of practice that you have always wanted to do but have never before had the opportunity. A number of registered practitioners are becoming very interested in alternative therapies, such as aromatherapy, massage or reflexology, either as a purely 'out-of-work activity' or as something that they think will enhance the care they can offer to patients and clients. Whatever you choose, it will take a lot of commitment and re-organization of your life and others around you.

Your objectives

Now that you have considered the options, you are ready to actually get your objectives down on paper. Although, for clarity, I have divided then up here, in reality you will probably find considerable overlap between them. It is likely to be helpful to think of them in terms of the short, medium and long term. Ideally they should include a mixture of things, to save having to do this exercise several times – in other words, they should be designed to meet your PREP objectives, meet your work objectives and meet your career objectives. They are, of course, only suggestions as to possible shape, and will need to be be tailor-made for your own circumstances. If you have done something like this before, you may well have your own way of setting things out, but if not, you might like to try the following.

Short term objectives (year 1). For the first year it is worth starting with something very straightforward, and it may look something like this:

1. Buy a folder to use as a personal professional profile.
2. Customize it within 3 months of purchase, to include at least:
   a. the PREP Fact sheets and/or the UKCC booklet 'PREP and You'

    b. your curriculum vitae

    c. your objectives for meeting the PREP requirements during the 3 years in question.

3. Decide roughly how you are going to meet your PREP objectives.
4. Complete at least one of your PREP days.
5. Obtain information on what managerial, clinical, academic or professional courses are available locally and decide what you might want to do. Your medium- and particularly your long-term objectives will influence your choice of activity here.

Medium term objectives (years 2-3)

1. Complete at least 3 PREP days in the second year.
2. Complete the fifth PREP day in the third year.
3. Undertake a short course on the principles of teaching (this may be the means of meeting objectives 1 and 2).
4. Apply for promotion to F grade post when one becomes available.
5. Start qualifying as an aromatherapist (this may also meet objectives 1 and 2, if you will be using the new skills at work).

Long term objectives (years 3–6). These will be very personal and could look something like:

1. Be managing your own team within 3 years, or
2. Commence a PhD within 4 years, or
3. Be at home raising a family within 6 years
4. Set up your own business as an aromatherapist within 6 years
5. Be working as a Trust chief executive within 3 years, or
6. Retire and start working in the voluntary sector within 7 years.

Objectives should always be flexible and should be reviewed on a regular basis depending on individual circumstances. 'Old' objectives are often a source of interest, if not amusement, when viewed with the longer lens of hindsight. As a student, my main objective was to be the sister of a gynaecological ward, mainly because that was my first 'ward' and I had some wonderful role models there. I didn't ever get anywhere near one, though, once I qualified!

I am sure you are getting the message. None of this is difficult and indeed you have probably been doing something similar for some time, even if you haven't thought about it in quite such an explicit way before – and you may well not have committed your thoughts to paper before. Try to think of your personal professional profile a bit like a diary that you can 'chat' to – it doesn't have to be written out in beautiful prose and spell-checked.

Recording what you have done

This is the part that is worrying a lot of people – how they fill in their personal professional profile. How much or how little to write. Will the UKCC be 'inspecting' the contents. Will there be rules for completion and what happens if it is not 'good enough'. I think that the main message is – don't worry. The UKCC have deliberately left the detail flexible at this stage. As I said earlier, more detailed guidance will be given over time, as evaluation take place of what has been done so far and the audit tools are piloted. But until such time as that further guidance or information appears, then follow the information in the fact sheets (UKCC 1994) and the *PREP and You* booklet (UKCC 1997), in terms of how much and what type of data to collect.

The main thing as far as undertaking any PREP activity is concerned is that you set objectives for each piece of activity – which is likely to be the individual day of study activity – and then record in your profile how that activity contributed to your professional practice. You don't have to write a lot – half a page of A4 may well be enough. But it needs to be enough so that you remember the event. You can identify the things that you learnt as a result; and you can describe how that will be relevant to maintaining and developing your knowledge and understanding.

First of all, though, *get started*. Think of all the energy that you are wasting worrying about it. That energy and time could be channelled into actually doing it. This would serve two useful purposes – it would stop you waking up in the night thinking, 'What am I going to do about that blankety-blank profile?' and it would also give you a sense of satisfaction that you have least started to crack it.

Above all, enjoy it. See lifelong learning as a privilege, not a chore. See it as a positive activity which helps to keep us up-to-date, which widens our horizons, which gives us new knowledge and skills, which improves the care that we give to our patients and clients, which gives us new things to talk about with family and friends and which is sure to make us even more interesting human beings.

HAPPY LEARNING!

REFERENCES

Howe G 1995 Conflict of loyalty. Macmillan, London
National Committee of Enquiry into Higher Education 1997a Higher education and the learning society (Dearing report). HMSO, London
National Committee of Enquiry into Higher Education 1997b Higher education in the learning society – the report of the Scottish committee (Garrick report). HMSO, Norwich
Nursing Times 1997 Stretched to breaking point (no named author). Insight. Nursing Times 9(29):
UKCC 1994 PREP fact sheets. UKCC, London (out of print)
UKCC 1997 PREP and you. UKCC, London

Appendices

CONTENTS

Appendix 1: your questions answered

INTRODUCTION

This appendix may become your favourite place in the book! It contains all the questions you have ever wanted to ask about PREP but thought they were too 'silly', 'obvious', or 'simple' to ask. These are words that have been used by other people when talking to me about PREP – they are certainly not mine. I have always been of the view that there is no such thing as a 'silly' question as far as PREP is concerned. If you, as a practitioner whose registration is affected by the PREP requirements don't know the answer, then that makes it a legitimate question. It could be, of course – indeed, I sincerely hope so – that the answer is already written down somewhere. It may just be that you have not yet been able to find the information that you want.

All the questions or statements here are ones that have been asked, or made, by real practitioners – at conferences, in letters, in personal telephone calls, through the PREP helpline, or to the professional press. I assure you that they have not been made up – although you might think that about some of them.

Together with the answer, the reader is also referred to that part of the text where the issue is discussed in more detail. As far as possible the questions are grouped together under the relevant broad subject area.

PRACTISING/IN PRACTICE
What...?

Q: I am working as a clinical services manager. Is that practising, in PREP terms?
A: Yes. If you are using your qualification in some capacity in your daily work, which I am sure you would be.

Q: Please clarify an argument we have been having at work. I say that PREP covers all sorts of nurses, but my friends say that it only applies to those who are in hands-on clinical practice.
A: It's really good to be right sometimes, isn't it? PREP is for all those using their nursing, midwifery or health visiting qualification in some capacity. It is definitely not only for those in clinical practice, although this was a common misconception, certainly in the early days.

Q: I qualified as a registered mental nurse before I became a policeman. Can I stay on the register under PREP?
A: Probably not, unless you are in a role where you are actually using your nursing qualifications on a regular basis, e.g. in a designated counselling role.

Where...?

Q: I have been working overseas for VSO for the last 4 years. Does that count? My friend said that I could only count it if I was working in the UK.
A: Friends aren't always right. 'Practice' can be undertaken anywhere, providing you are using your nursing, midwifery or health visiting qualification in some capacity. There is nothing in PREP which says where you have to be practising.

Mind you, it's an easy mistake to make because overseas experience used not to be given much credit by employers. And it still does not count towards your 'continuous' service for employment/pension purposes.

Q: I have an RMNH qualification and am employed by social services. Can I still keep my registration?
A: Yes, providing that you are using it in your work. It doesn't matter if the previous post holder was not a nurse, as long as you feel that you use your qualification to give quality care.

When...?

Q: Do I have to do my practice hours evenly across the 5 year period?
A: No, fit them in as you like. They could be done in one 'lump', either at the beginning or at the end of the period, or spread throughout the whole time. But don't forget to keep a record of the hours you work in your personal professional profile, otherwise you will never remember them!

Q: I have worked on nights for the last 20 years and don't want to change. My manager says that PREP says you have to work at least 100 working days in every 5 year period. She says that means I have to do internal rotation of day and night duty.
A: It is true that PREP says that a break in practice is defined as 'working for 100 working days or less'. That is not, however, meant to be taken literally. A working 'day' can definitely include night duty.

Q: I am working in a nurse bank and do between 8 and 36 hours a month. I'm not sure how this fits in with the return to practice requirements. Can you help please?
A: The most important thing to remember is to keep a record of the hours that you work in your personal professional profile, then you can use that information to work it out. From the year 2000, you have to do a statutory return to practice course if you have done less than 100 working days or 750 hours in the previous 5 year period. If you have only been doing 8 hours a month, then in 5 years you will have done 480 hours and would need to do a return to practice course. However, if you were doing 36 hours a month, you will have clocked up 2160 hours, so you wouldn't need to do anything more. Remember you can do the hours at any time, so if you see yourself getting short of the number of hours towards the end of the 5 year period, you might want to increase the hours you are doing, if that is possible.

Q: Where do I get details of return to practice courses from?
A: The National Board in the country where you want to do the course. The addresses are in Appendix 2.

Why...?

Q: I think that all the PREP requirements are bureaucratic rubbish. I trained years ago at a very prestigious training school and I don't see why I should have to keep up-to-date.
A: I hope you are not on duty the night I'm admitted.

How...?

Q: I have had to give up work to look after my father-in-law, who has had a stroke. I am only 45 and want to come back to work as soon as I can and I don't want to lose my registration.
A: I have good news for you. If you are in a situation where you are using your qualification, even though you are not waged, then you can count that as 'practice' as far as PREP is concerned, providing you meet certain criteria. See pages 112–113 for details.

Q: I am not currently employed as a nurse in a hospital. However, I am a nursing officer in the Red Cross. Does that count for PREP purposes?
A: Certainly, providing you are doing enough hours. See page 132 for definition of a break in practice.

LAPSED REGISTRATION

Q: Please help. I've just realized that my registration has lapsed. My manager says that I am to be suspended.
A: Don't panic, but you do need to take action as quickly as possible. You

need to contact the registration department at the UKCC as a matter of urgency. If you have been lapsed for more than 3 months, you will need to provide three references supporting your application, as well as pay your fee and complete a NoP form. If it is less than that, you only have to pay your fee and complete a NoP form. If you have been lapsed less than 3 months, it will take 5 days to get re-registered, if you are quick about sending in the necessary information. If you have been lapsed for longer than 3 months, then it will take 7–10 days depending on how quickly you can get your references to the UKCC. Faxing them in speeds up the process, of course.

The sanction that your manager takes is up to him/her, although if it has been made clear to employees what the sanctions are for practising without being registered, then you probably can't expect much sympathy. Have a word with your professional organization or trade union, if necessary.

Q: I am letting my registration lapse because I don't see why I should have to meet these bureaucratic requirements.
A: That is your right, although I don't agree with you. As a matter of accuracy, PREP is not, of course, about bureaucratic requirements, but about maintaining and developing professional knowledge and competence. However, if you do decide to let your registration lapse, it does mean that you would not be eligible for employment in a position requiring a registered nurse. If you are currently employed, to let your registration lapse would be very unwise, as employers can, and do, use severe sanctions against such individuals (see p. 134).

Q: My employer has just told me that, as my registration has lapsed, I will be paid as an auxiliary until it has been renewed. Can they do that?
A: In a word, yes… Renewing your registration is your business. Employers are known to take a range of sanctions if they discover that someone's registration has lapsed. The sanctions can vary from suspension without pay, suspension with pay, payment as an auxiliary, employing a registered practitioner to shadow you until your registration is renewed, to dismissal.

Q: I have decided to retire early. Whilst I agree with the idea of PREP, I really don't have the energy to start studying again at my age.
A: Don't rush into the decision without being sure of your facts. It would certainly be worth renewing your registration for the first time it falls due after 1 April 1995, as all you have to do is pay your fee and complete a NoP form. By the end of that period you only have to have completed 5 days of study activity, which you may well be doing already. Re-read PREP fact sheet 3 to see how flexible it can be. The final decision is yours, of course.

Q: What is the upper age limit for registration with the Council?
A: There isn't one.

STUDY ACTIVITY

Q: I have been told that I have to choose a study day from each of the five categories.
A: Not true. Choose all five of your days from one category if you wish, or mix them up – it's up to you.

Q: Where do I get details of approved study days?
A: Nowhere, because there are no PREP 'approved' study days (see next section).

Q: How do I find out what's available, in terms of the sort of study activity I could choose from, to meet my PREP?
A: You will be spoilt for choice. See Appendix 3 for details.

Q: My manager says that I have to do the days she has chosen for me.
A: Not so. The choice is up to you. However, if you want as much support as possible, it might be worth seeing what sort of compromises can be made – how about you doing two of the days that are suggested, if they are relevant, and negotiating for your own choice on the others? With a bit of tact, diplomacy and luck, you will probably both be happy.

Q: I am doing a course on reflexology at the moment. Can I count that for PREP purposes?
A: Yes, if you are going to use the skills at work.

Q: I can't afford to spend money on expensive study days. I can only just manage as it is, but I can't possibly afford to lose my registration.
A: A lot of people are in a situation similar to the one you describe. That is one of the reasons why the UKCC made the achieving of the requirements so flexible. You *don't* have to spend a lot of money to complete your PREP requirements. Why not get together with some friends/colleagues in someone's house to discuss current professional issues. Providing you have objectives for the session and record the outcomes in your profile, you will have met the requirements and probably enjoyed yourselves as well – all for the cost of some coffee and biscuits.

Q: Can I 'collect up' shorter periods of study activity to make up a whole PREP day?
A: Yes, a good idea. For example, if you attend a series of evening lectures over, say, 5 or 6 weeks, then together that would make up the equivalent of a whole day.

Approval of study days

Q: I am totally confused about approved study days.
A: You're not the only one. There is a lot of misinformation about! From the

horse's mouth – *there are no such things as approved PREP study days*. The choice of study activity, whether it be in the form of a study day or some other type of activity, is entirely up to you. If you see something advertised as 'PREP approved' then please let the UKCC know and they will take it up with the advertising organization/person concerned. However, you may well see something advertised which suggests that you might 'use this to meet your PREP requirements'. That's fine because it leaves the decision with you as to whether it is suitable or not, to meet your particular needs.

Q: I have accumulated a lot of continuing education points (CEPs). Can I use these on their own to prove to the UKCC that I have met my PREP requirements?
A: No. The UKCC recognizes no points systems as evidence in their own right of continuing education. However, provided that you have kept a record of what you got the CEPs for – and have recorded in your profile how that study contributed to your professional practice – then that's fine.

NOTIFICATION OF PRACTICE FORM

Q: I think the notification of practice form is just bureaucracy gone mad. I'm not going to bother to fill mine in.
A: That is a great shame, then, as it means your registration will lapse and you will not be able to practise as a registered nurse, midwife or health visitor. Completing the form is an integral part of the legislative requirements for registration – not an optional extra.

Q: I don't think the notification of practice form is very accurate. I work overseas and it doesn't have a special section for that.
A: I agree that the NoP form isn't perfect, but it can't accommodate every type of nursing, midwifery and community practice, or it would go on for pages and pages. The UKCC has tried to make its categories as comprehensive as possible, but there will always be those who don't quite 'fit' – hence there will always be a need for an 'other' category. In your particular case, I don't think that practising overseas is a separate category of practice, in its own right, but a geographical location – it is the type of practice that is important. I agree, however, that it would be useful for the Council's statistics to know, in addition to knowing the type of practice, whether someone was working in the UK or abroad, and if so, where. The NoP form is reviewed on a regular basis and this can be considered as part of the next review.

Q: The NoP form is just a ruse on the part of the Government to get private details about the movements of qualified nurses and midwives, so that they can reduce the numbers of trained staff.
A: We're all entitled to our own views – but you're wrong, on two counts. First, the UKCC is set up as an entirely independent organization, financed by registrants, with no formal government links. Second, information from

the UKCC's register is available to everyone, either in the published annual statistics or on written request, providing that it meets the criteria for the use of the register, which is publicly available from the Council.

SPECIALIST PRACTICE

Q: I am a practice nurse and my friend said that the UKCC say that I have to have a specialist qualification by October 1998 or I will lose my job.
A: Your friend has got her/his facts wrong. The UKCC does not require anyone to have to get a specialist qualification. An employer may think that it is a good idea, but if so, they would have to have discussed it with you. It could not retrospectively be made a requirement for the job, unless that had been made part of your job offer, at interview.

Q: I've done loads of study days in my time, although I don't believe in all this certificate collecting. I think I should be able to get a specialist qualification without doing any more work.
A: That, regrettably, is not possible. Things which are worth getting usually require some more work and this is no exception. The best thing to do first, if you do decide that you do want to find out about getting a specialist qualification, is to contact one of the National Boards. Their addresses can be found in Appendix 2.

Q: I am an SRN and I've been working as a practice nurse for 10 years. I haven't done any courses since qualification. Can I call myself a specialist practitioner?
A: No. Not in the definition adopted by the UKCC. See page 142 for more details.

Q: Where can I get details about getting a specialist qualification?
A: Start with your National Board. It would also be worth seeing what your local university/higher education college has available.

Q: Where can I get funding to do a specialist course?
A: It depends where you are working and what the arrangements are for funding courses. In the first instance, find out whether your employer is prepared to support you in doing the course and, if so, whether that involves financial support. Then see if he/she knows about the funding available in your Trust. The National Boards will also be able to give you some advice. If you are working as a practice nurse, the best person to talk to would be the nurse adviser at the health authority. Your local higher education institution may also have information about sources of funding.

PERSONAL PROFESSIONAL PROFILE

Q: I can't afford to spend a lot on my profile.

A: That's OK. There is no reason why you should have to. No-one is ever going to be judging the quality of the container. Why not buy an ordinary ring binder from the newsagents.

Q: My manager wants me to use my PREP profile as part of my annual appraisal.
A: That's quite a complex issue. The main thing is that the profile is your own personal property and no-one else has access to all of its contents without your permission. See pages 129–130 where this is discussed in more detail.

Q: I'm terrified at the thought of having to do my profile. Where on earth do I start?
A: Don't worry – lots of people feel just the same as you do. Start by reading PREP fact sheet no. 4 (UKCC 1994), or the UKCC booklet *PREP and you* (UKCC 1997). There are also a lot of books on the market now which look at profiles in more detail, which can be really helpful. Why not get together with a friend who is also worried and get started together?

Q: I've been told that if I attend a PREP lecture, I have to write the whole thing out in full in my personal professional profile.
A: Not so. It's not the content of the session that is the important thing – it's how it helped you to maintain and develop your professional practice. So you would only want a brief synopsis of the content and then a commentary on what you did as a result of this increased knowledge.

Q: I've been told that UKCC officers will have the power to visit our places of work and could demand to 'inspect' our profiles.
A: I've heard that one as well! It's amazing what people will believe – but that really is the equivalent of the stories that are made up to frighten little children... No truth in it whatsoever.

MIDWIFERY

Q: I've been told that PREP does not affect midwives, as they already have their own legislation about refresher courses.
A: Not true. Yes, it is correct that midwives have had legislation relating to refresher course for a long time (Rule 37). This legislation has now been incorporated into the PREP rules. From 2001 all those on the register – nurse, midwife or health visitor – will have to meet the same requirements. See pages 132–133 for more details.

Q: Do I still have to do courses approved by a National Board? We've had to do this for so long, I can't believe that it doesn't apply any longer.
A: You have a choice until 2001. If you want to do a course that is put on by a National Board, then that's fine, but you don't have to. The NBs are not required to go on providing them after 2001 but may decide to do so, and it's up to the individuals if they want to choose something of their own, or something provided by a Board.

Q: Why do I have to complete a notification of intention to practise form and a notification of practice form? Surely that is duplication of information and my effort.
A: Good point, but they are actually designed for different things. The notification of intention to practise form is part of the legislative requirements associated with midwifery supervision. The notification of practice form is part of the PREP requirements for maintaining registration.

Q: Do I still have to come to the UK to complete a refresher course?
A: No. You can choose something relevant wherever you are working.

Q: Do I have to practise in the UK to 'get my hours in' for PREP?
A: No. PREP makes no statements about where you need to be practising.

USE OF TITLE

Q: I am very proud of my SRN qualification and don't want to lose it. Can I go on using it? I'm not working any longer.
A: It's quite understandable to be proud of a qualification for which you worked so hard. Providing there is no intent to deceive people into thinking you are eligible for practice as a registered nurse, midwife or health visitor, then you can use the qualification, e.g. on letterheads and so on. See page 135 for details.

RETIREMENT

Q: I'm due to retire next December and my registration is due for renewal in March that year. Is it worth all the hassle of renewing it?
A: You need to make a decision according to your personal circumstances. For the first time of renewal after 1 April 1995, it would be worth renewing, as all you have to do is pay the fee and complete the NoP from. That gives you 3 years' 'grace' by the end of which you must have completed the study activity. Two years after that if you are still not practising, then your registration will lapse anyway because you won't meet the hours of practice requirements. If there is any chance that you may still continue to practise in any way that may need your registration, then keep meeting the requirements – it's easier to maintain registration than to have to renew it.

REFERENCES

UKCC 1993 Midwives rules. UKCC, London
UKCC 1994 PREP fact sheets. UKCC, London (out of print)
UKCC 1997 PREP and you. UKCC, London

Appendix 2: sources of information

This appendix links to Chapter 6 and gives some suggestions as to where you might like to seek information about courses, study days, study activity and so on.

National Boards for Nursing, Midwifery and Health Visiting

The National Boards for Nursing, Midwifery and Health Visiting in each country of the UK will provide information on the professional courses that they approve.

Pre-registration programmes

Courses leading to registration in:
- midwifery
- health visiting
- adult nursing
- mental health nursing
- learning disabilities nursing
- children's nursing.

Post-registration courses

Programmes leading to:
- specialist qualifications in a range of different areas of practice, e.g. health visiting/public health nursing or critical care nursing
- teaching qualifications
- supervisor of midwives' qualifications
- registration on another part of the register.

Addresses
English National Board for Nursing, Midwifery and Health Visiting
Victory House
170 Tottenham Court Road
London
W1P 0HA

NBS – National Board for Nursing, Midwifery and Health Visiting for Scotland
22 Queen Street
Edinburgh
EH2 1JT

Northern Ireland National Board for Nursing, Midwifery and Health Visiting
Centre House
79 Chichester Street
Belfast
BT1 4JE

Welsh National Board for Nursing, Midwifery and Health Visiting
Second floor
Golate House
101 St Mary Street
Cardiff
CF1 1DX

Professional organizations/trade unions

Many professional organizations offer an excellent range of services, including study days, conferences, distance learning and continuing education activities, for both members and others. Activities will always be cheaper for members, but are often reasonably priced anyway. Each organization provides a range of information on what they have to offer. Individual special interest groups within the wider organization may also provide subject specific material.

Royal College of Nursing
20 Cavendish Square
London
W1M 0AB

RCN Continuing Education Office
RCN Institute of Advanced Nursing Education
20 Cavendish Square
London
W1M 0AB

Royal College of Midwives
14 Mansfield Street
London
W1M 0BE

Publications/Continuing Education Department
Royal College of Midwives
4 Cathedral Road
Cardiff
CF1 9LJ

Community Practitioner and Health Visitors Association
50 Southwark Street
London
SE1 1UN

Queen's Nursing Institute
3 Albermarle Way
Clerkenwell
London
EC1V 4JB

Medical Defence Union – Publications
192 Altrincham Road
Manchester
M22 4RZ

UNISON Education and Training
Civic House
20 Grand Depot Road
London
SE18 6SF

Universities/institutes of higher education

Information on:

- access courses
- first degrees
- masters degrees
- doctorates
- diplomas/certificates.

Addresses: local libraries, UCAS handbook.

Distance learning centres

Information may also be obtained from:

Macmillan Open Learning
Professional Practice Study Units
Porter's South
Crinan Street
London
N1 9XW

The Open Learning Foundation
3 Devonshire Street
London
W1N 2BA

The Open University
PO Box 724
Walton Hall
Milton Keynes
MK7 6ZS

Further education colleges

Information on vocational courses such as:

- complementary therapies
- computing skills
- practical teaching skills course, e.g. City and Guilds 730 Further Education Teacher's Certificate
- return to study skills.

Addresses: local telephone directories, local library.

Your own institution

An increasing number of trusts, hospitals, nursing homes and so on are starting to put on continuing education events for staff. These can range from short, subject-specific lectures to longer courses on a variety of work-based issues. What is on offer will usually have been designed to meet the particular needs of the specific institution. You may also be able to have access to what's available at neighbouring institutions.

Shared learning/other organizations

Don't forget to check what is being offered by other professions in the way of CPD that might be suitable. All the professions supplementary to medicine and doctors will be doing some sort of continuing education of some sort or another, not to mention those working outside the health care setting. Sharing educational experiences with other professions is frequently a very interesting way of gaining a broader perspective on multiprofessional issues. In many cases, it is essential in terms of improving the quality of the care available to patients and clients. Some likely interprofessional combinations might be:

- practice nurses, district nurses and general practitioners
- midwives and obstetricians
- health visitors, social workers and the police
- community psychiatric nurses and psychiatric social workers
- specialist nurses and their medical counterparts
- rehabilitation nurses and physiotherapists.

The possibilities are endless!

There are also a range of other organizations that may well provide events that would be of great interest and relevance. Organizations such as the Patient's Association, the Consumer's Association or the Association of Community Health Councils, to name but a few, are very likely to have events from which many health care professionals would benefit.

Professional press

The professional press is a rich source of information on a range of learning activities and several of them also provide personal profiles. The only problem is that the information on continuing education tends to be in those inserts that fall out and spread themselves all over the newsagents floor when you open the journal – or worse, if you get to them second or third hand, they have already disappeared. Don't throw them away if you drop them and try and find them if they have disappeared – they are worth looking at. There are adverts for:

- educational courses
- study days on every conceivable subject
- study programmes
- conferences
- individual articles on virtually every subject.

Some words of warning

Just a word of warning. If the only part of the book that you are reading is this appendix and you may therefore have missed it elsewhere – don't be misled by the implication given by some advertisers that their activity is 'PREP approved'. Remember, *you* are the person who decides what is relevant to you. There is no such thing as central approval from any organization – and certainly not from the UKCC. Be cautious about what is on offer and use your 'purchasing power' wisely. Remember, a register of 640 000 registrants is a very lucrative market for education providers and there are always those willing to exploit the gullible. You, as an intelligent, accountable professional, must check things out for yourself.

What should you look for? These are the sorts of general questions that you would want to ask:

- *What do you know about the organization offering the course?* Is it an accredited HE or FE educational institution or a professional organization/ trades union? If so, then you can be reasonably sure that you are being offered a 'quality product'. You also have someone to complain to if you are not happy.

If, on the other hand, you have not heard of the organization/company offering the activity, you will want to be more cautious. It may be that this is purely a commercial organization with little knowledge of the health/ education service. Ask around – has anyone heard of it, or been to previous events they have run? How much are they charging? What are you getting for your money?

- *Has the course been validated by a National Board for Nursing, Midwifery or Health Visiting?* If so, you know that you have a 'quality benchmark' already in place.

- *Has the course been validated by any other national body, such as CETSW or the British Psychological Society, for example?* If so, you should be assured of a quality product.

- *Are the objectives of the event (whether it be a study day or a course) clear, measurable and relevant to your own professional requirements?* They should be, because otherwise, how do you know what you are 'buying'? You certainly won't know at the end of the day whether any objectives have been met, if they haven't been made explicit in advance.

- *What are the qualifications and experience of those to whom you will be listening? Do they know their stuff?* Check what is said about the speakers. Does it look as though they will know what they are talking about? What evidence is being offered by way of proof. Beware of phases like 'a wealth of experience' or 'years in the business' if no corroborating evidence is given.

- *What supplementary material will you receive, such as abstracts or resumes of the speakers papers?* Such information is always useful and will help remind you what the sessions were about in due course.

- *What about certificates of attendance?* Not necessary, in PREP terms, as it's your profile entry about the event that matters, rather than just the bald record of you having been somewhere. Also, some events hand out the certificates as you go in, thus providing no proof of anything other than your having collected the certificate! On the other hand, I have a suspicion that most of us quite like having something to show for the event and it will help remind you of what you've done. So, providing that the 'certificate' is not the only thing in your PPP in relation to the activity, then why not?

- *What if the event turns out to be poor value?* Providing that you have taken reasonable steps to check things out, this is hardly your fault. In terms of PREP you need to look for the things that *were* helpful – like meeting people during the lunch break or following up some new ideas. After all, you aren't going to want to do another day, just because this one didn't deliver. But make sure that your expectations were reasonable and check out the reality of the event against the publicity material. If you genuinely think that the organizers didn't deliver what they promised then do write and tell them – they won't know unless you do. Do it as a separate letter – not just on the evaluation form because that can get lost amongst a mass of others.

Appendix 3: ways of meeting your PREP requirements and what they say about PREP

INTRODUCTION

The purpose of this appendix is to look at what is available for meeting the PREP requirements. Let me stress again, as I have throughout the book, that the *choice* of what you do is your decision and yours alone. However, you may find it helpful to see what's available on the general market (Section A) and also what some individuals are doing, or planning to do, to meet the requirements (Section B). I think that a lot of people find it easier to get their own ideas off the ground once someone has given them a few hints – I know that I do.

The following information is set out so that you can make informed judgements as to what meets your needs. I offer no comment on the relative quality or suitability of the offerings – it all depends on what suits you, your style of learning, the time you have available, your pocket, and so on. The activities are set out in no order of preference. I would suggest that you might like to use the questions set out in Appendix 2 on sources of information as a framework to assess the suitability of what's on offer at any time.

SECTION A

Professional press

The professional press will provide a rich source of information on a number of continuing professional development activities. They will, of course, in the main, have a cost attached but I hope that the information given below will confirm for you that there is great benefit to be had from shopping around. I have included the cost of the event on offer, where that information was included, merely to demonstrate the diversity. One of the journals, for example, runs a series of three × 2 day conferences throughout the UK each year and they are free, including a range of presentations from expert speakers together with a huge professional exhibition – absolutely unbeatable value. Just a quick scan through the journals will give you a number of suggestions that you might like to consider.

Conferences/study days

A random trawl through two or three professional journals only, in one week in September 1997, showed the following activities being advertised.

International conferences on:

- Clinical trials and ethics (Belgium)
- Evidence-based child health nursing (Jersey)
- Nurse practitioner conference (Australia)
- The psychosocial impacts of breast cancer (Switzerland)
- Empowerment and health – an agenda for nurses in the 21st century (Brunei).

National conferences on:

- Current policy and practice (£80/£100)
- Private concern – public accountability – surgical intervention for children (£73/£99)
- VQs and their impact on nursing (£75/£100)
- Evidence based nursing – wound care (£55/£80)
- Working with families (£75/£115)
- Breaking the barriers – challenging current midwifery practice (£35)
- A vision for healthcare – 2000 and beyond (no cost given)
- Exploring developments in gynaecological cancer, the menopause and HRT (£60/£75)
- Looking to the future – outpatient nurses (£65/£75)
- Infection control (£75/£85)
- Wound care master class (no cost given)
- Genetics and the midwife (£545 residential £423 non-residential)
- Black and minority ethnic women NHS managers and professionals (no cost given)
- Acute pain management (£123)
- Research and the Midwife (£45)
- Nurse led primary care (£110/£130)
- Effectively managing information (£90)
- Psychosocial medicine in practice (£130).

(Where two prices are given, that reflects the difference between either members/ non-members of the organisation offering the event or subscribers/non-subscribers of the organising journal.)

Local conferences/study days on :

- Pregnancy nutrition (£15)
- Colorectal cancer (£25)
- Evidenced-based midwifery practice (£47)
- Promoting patient-centred practice (free)
- Violence against women (£60)
- Emergency care (£20)
- Mental health in children's nursing (no cost details)
- Working with postnatal depression – a mother's perspective (£70)
- Acute pain (£30)
- Focus on women's health (£35)
- Home birth in practice.

This small and random sample demonstrates very clearly the range and cost of study activity. The geographical spread of the events was also wide, ranging all over the UK and beyond. There is a clear message here – shop around. Study days are likely to be much cheaper than conferences as they will have fewer overheads. They can, however, be equally good value and many people prefer smaller, more interactive events.

Courses

In the same week, the same journals also advertised the following courses (long and short). No cost information was included in the advertisements:

- Managing safety in the NHS
- Counselling skills and theory training
- Bachelor of midwifery (Hons)
- MSc in care, policy and management
- Prevention and secondary care of the breast cancer patient
- Ophthalmic nursing course (ENB 346)
- MSc in complementary medicine
- Understanding ageing and older people.

This sample is not intended to be exhaustive – there were also lots of other events. It has, I hope, however, served my purpose of demonstrating that there is a vast range of activity on offer. And we haven't finished yet!

Distance learning

Many of the professional journals now offer – either individually or in conjunction with another organization – some excellent distance learning materials. These usually include some form of printed material on a specific topic and often incorporate a variety of different media. They are often supplemented by some form of assessment. The assessment is not required for PREP purposes, but individuals may prefer to have a formal route for the assessment of their knowledge. Most of the materials will indicate which of the PREP study 'categories' are accommodated by the particular piece of learning activity. Write to the individual journals themselves for more information.

Professional organizations

Professional organizations are usually assiduous in their provision of high-quality continuing education offerings. Not only do they arrange a wide and varied range of conferences on professional issues, which are invariably cheaper for members, but they often also provide other activity. Distance learning materials using a range of media, such as television, CD-ROMs, tapes, and so on, are imaginatively produced and can be used at any time of day or night, which may be a great advantage to some users.

Statutory bodies

The statutory bodies increasingly provide a range of 'meet us' days or conferences, designed to discuss specific or general professional issues. The UKCC works hard to honour its UK role and has professional conferences throughout the four countries. The National Boards offer events in their own countries and such events are often available to those from any part of the UK.

SECTION B

In this section, I have set out a number of real examples and quotations from individual practitioners who have already decided what they are going to do to meet their requirements, in whole or in part. The sources of the information vary, from direct contact with those who have spoken or written to me or to colleagues, to experiences written up in the professional press. Again, no judgement is offered as to what is more or less suitable – these are things that suit the individuals concerned.

What real people are doing

'I have arranged a series of visits to recovery wards as I feel that is an area in which I need to expand her knowledge'. (Staff nurse – theatres)

'I am running a club – after work – for all those who want to come to discuss professional issues. It's free and there is a lot of interest. Midwives "collect up" the hours to make study days.' (Senior midwife manager)

'I am going to do a return to practice course because I've been out of practice for some time and it's a good way of getting up to date. I know that it's not actually a legislative requirement yet, but I think it's a good thing to do.' (Staff nurse – outpatients)

'I am attending several study days organized by the professional journals and I am preparing some papers on a new topic (that is, new to me) for publication.' (Nurse consultant)

'I am watching *Casualty* on TV. It is one of the few well researched medical dramas, with three professional advisers, a nurse, a doctor and a paramedic. I've learnt about the Alexander technique and updated my cardiac resuscitation techniques after watching Charlie defibrillate a patient in asystole and then having done some supplementary reading.' (Staff Nurse)

'We're doing a job swap for 2 months. It helps us get to know each other's areas of practice and expands our own skills.' (F grade sisters in A&E and Intensive care)

'I am reading and reflecting on a series of articles in the professional journals relevant to my particular area of clinical interest.' (Nurse lecturer)

What they've said about PREP

The following quotations are taken from an article entitled 'Are nurses prepared for PREP' in the *Nursing Standard* (Waters 1997). I thought they provided a very representative selection of the things that are said about PREP – warts and all.

I would be very surprised if you don't find something to identify with here:

'My portfolio is finished because I was applying for a G grade post. It was a really good exercise because it makes you reflect on your career.' (Ward Manager – vascular/high dependency unit)

'For what we get paid and the way we get treated, I think it's a real cheek to make us do all this extra work. I know we are accountable, but we need more incentives to do it. Otherwise it's just another hassle.' (Staff nurse)

'I have a folder (profile) because we were encouraged to keep one on my conversion course, but I don't believe many nurses panic about it because it's not many study days. I'd like to see more wards supply information and a supervision system incorporated into PREP.' (Recently converted enrolled nurse)

'I don't have a profile yet but I'll be able to put one together fairly easily. It's those nurses who qualified years ago and have stayed in their posts for years, that's where PREP is aimed at. Also for agency nurses. Sometimes I think, when did they train?' (Ward manager, oncology)

'Some people have done a lot for PREP and others have done nothing. It should be common sense but doesn't seem to be working that way. Some nurses find it difficult to study and they need encouragement.' (Practice development sister)

'Personally I think PREP is not enough. Five study days in 3 years is not sufficient to keep anyone up to date.' (Ward manager, oncology)

'There are so many dodgy nurses, some are really, really worrying. Hopefully PREP will weed those out, although I'm not sure it is an effective way of keeping up standards. Anyone can write a load of rubbish down.' (Staff nurse)

'Some have shown me profiles which are inches thick but they have only been qualified a year. It shows that people don't understand it's about reflective practice.' (Practice development nurse)

And from some research done by Margaret Johnson (1993, 1994) on profiling:

'The ideas of keeping a work "diary" is all very well in theory but it's one of those things where you either like to do it or can't stand doing it.'

'Before I had a profile self-doubt was a problem, but now when I realize how much I've achieved when I see it written down, my confidence increases.'

'Generally I'm not impressed with having a profile. I'm 40 years old and have no aspirations to gain promotion. Therefore, apart from providing the UKCC with proof of regular updating, I have no need to actively practise personal profiling.'

'It makes me nervous because I don't know what it involves – also it sounds like hard work in an already busy life.'

'I think it's a good idea. It helps you to keep the grey matter grey. It will make us all alert to changes and capable of coping.'

'I still have a great deal of lethargy about it although I understand that it's useful.'

'It has increased my awareness and self-esteem.'

In a *Nursing Times* article, Chris Buswell (1997) estimates the cost of PREP in the following way:

The UKCC informs her (the newly qualified nurse) of the PREP requirements and in a fluster she signs up for her minimum five days of education this year, just in case she's too busy next year. Depending on her choice of study days, conferences or courses this may cost her between £90 and £500. However, it may be more. She's bought a profile pack to help her account for her PREP but she's not quite sure what to do with it. Not a bad investment for £23.'

Fortunately readers were neither as ill-informed or as defeatist as the writer and he is put firmly in his place by Suzanne Lee (1997) in the following letter in the same publication:

Mr Buswell warns us that to sign up for PREP will account for an estimated £90–£500 and £23 respectively – rubbish. Continuing education beyond registration can be free. A day in the library, as long as it is relevant and can be shown to contribute to practice, is acceptable. Also the study hours obtainable through the *Nursing Times* are a cheaper alternative at only £1 a week. As for profiles – make your own.

I couldn't have put it better myself – thank you Suzanne.

REFERENCES

Buswell C 1997 What do you pay to work? Nursing Times 93(38):
Johnson H M 1993 Developing a positive attitude to personal professional profiling. Project for MA(Ed), Oxford Brooks University, Oxford
Johnson H M 1994 Evaluating personal profiles. MA(Ed) dissertation, Oxford Brooks University, Oxford
Lee S 1997 Letters. Nursing Times 93(40): 22
Waters A 1997 Are nurses prepared for PREP. Nursing Standard 11(52): 12

Index